S0-BYZ-633

ABOUT FACE

5-5c

Beauty

225471

ABOUT FACE

by Lewis M. Feder, M.D.
and Jane MacLean Craig

WARNER BOOKS

A Time Warner Company

Acknowledgments

We would like to express our sincerest appreciation to two women whose astute guidance and invaluable support worked to make this book a reality—our literary agent, Elaine Markson, and our editor at Warner Books, Leslie Keenan.

LMF and JMC

In addition, I would like to offer my heartfelt thanks to my husband, Tom, and my two wonderful children, T.J. and MacLean, for their enduring patience and understanding; and especially to my late aunt Caie Carter; for their love and support.

JMC

The information contained in this book is not intended as a substitute for medical advice. You are advised to consult regularly with your health care professional in matters relating to your health, and particularly where diagnosis or medical attention may be required. The information presented in this book is accurate as of May, 1989.

Copyright © 1989 by Lewis M. Feder and Jane MacLean Craig
All rights reserved.

Warner Books, Inc., 666 Fifth Avenue, New York, NY 10103

W A Time Warner Company

Printed in the United States of America
First Printing: September 1989
10 9 8 7 6 5 4 3 2

Library of Congress Cataloging-in-Publication Data

Feder, Lewis M.
 About face / by Lewis M. Feder and Jane MacLean Craig.
  p. cm.
 ISBN 0-446-38992-7 (pbk.) (U.S.A.)
      0-446-38993-5 (pbk.) (Can.)
  1. Skin—Care and hygiene. I. Craig, Jane MacLean, c1954–   .
II. Title.
RL87.F43 1989
646.7'26—dc20

89-14670
CIP

Cover design by Victoria Peslak/Platinum Design
Cover photo by The Image Bank
Book design by Giorgetta Bell McRee

For my late father, Al,
for his warmth and
inspiration;
To my mother Gerrie;
And my wonderful sister Jane.

With My Love
LMF

Contents

Introduction

If I was asked to define the essence of world-class beauty, I would have to say it's beautiful skin—the first (and most impressive) facet of every first impression. Contrary to popular belief, beautiful skin is *not* something held in reserve for the rich and famous. It's an attribute attainable by anyone who knows a few simple, yet vitally important, "secrets." This invaluable information (which you're about to learn) will enable you to *erase six to twelve years* from your appearance in only ninety days.

To understand my confidence in making this claim, you must first gain a bit of insight on my particular area of medical expertise. As a specialist in the fields of cosmetic dermatology and cosmetic surgery ("appearance" medicine), my goal is to maximize each individual's potential for good looks. In so doing, I'm proud to say, I've earned an unprecedented reputation for success, attracting the most celebrated beauties of our time to my Manhattan practice. It was, in fact, in the process of meeting the rigorous demands associated with maintaining such high visibility that the skincare revolution you're about to discover was born.

After all, if your face really *is* your fortune, you can't afford to gamble with the condition of your skin. A highly visible woman needs a program of care on which she can rely unconditionally for consistently superlative results. And that's exactly what I've provided.

Introduction

Until now, the details of this extraordinary plan have been quietly guarded for the sole use of my private patients. But with this book, I'm able to share them with each of you, as well, enabling *you* to reap the rewards evidenced in the faces of those you've admired from afar!

Why My Approach Is Different

CHAPTER 1

If you're like most people, your interest in discovering a viable elixir of youth has probably grown stronger with each passing year. As time starts to etch in the skin a record of life's experiences, it's natural to long for a "miracle" to restore it to its wrinkle-free prime.

If you tend to believe what you read, you've undoubtedly become convinced that such a treasure—the pot of gold at the end of the rainbow, if you will—is as close as your nearest cosmetics counter. Why, then, in spite of diligently following every advertised route to instant beauty, haven't you been able to find it? The answer, sought by many a weary "rainbow chaser," lies in the age-old adage "You get what you pay for."

And what you paid for when you bought that high-priced lotion, potion, or creme was expensive (and effective) advertising, *not* skincare—and that's exactly what you got! After all, it brought you into the store a "believer," didn't it? Still, using these products gives rise to a disillusioning realization, and all too often a harmful effect on the skin, ultimately costing much more than the purchase price. Take the case of Sara V.

A prominent New York socialite, Sara was what I term a victim of the "mature skincare syndrome." Although still oily-skinned, her age (between 35 and 40) indicated to an overzealous (and grossly undertrained) department store "beauty advisor" that she was a candidate for a regimen geared to the mature or dry-skinned individual. Unfortunately, Sara fell prey to her insecurities.

Intended for *very* dry skin (a condition that has nothing to do with one's chronological age), the program she was advised to buy consisted of one superemollient, lanolin-rich creme on top of another. After several weeks of daily applications, Sara discovered—to her chagrin—that her $200 purchase had also cost her her blemish-free complexion!

She was more than mildly disheartened when she came to me for help. I let her know that she was not, by any means, the first (or the last) to make such a mistake. I couldn't begin to count the number of patients who, feeling a bit frightened about the onset of wrinkles, have found themselves in exactly the same situation.

I ordered an immediate halt to all of Sara's newly acquired skincare products and recommended she undertake the program of care I have designed for the oily-skinned individual. A brewer's yeast mask applied three times per week, as well as daily application of a grapefruit/vodka/mineral water toner (both described in Part I), greatly aided in the healing of her blemishes.

Sara has remained on my program of suggested care and has a beautiful, wrinkle-free complexion to show for it today. After experimenting with virtually every skincare line in existence, Sara is now an ardent fan of my natural approach.

Unfortunately, many other women will be caught up in the cosmetics industry's web of deception. Why? Because there is a third certainty, of almost equal weight with death and taxes, and cosmetics manufacturers know they can count on it ad infinitum: *There will always be a buyer for hope.* Thus, each new season brings with it their latest waves of entries, additions to a sea already overflowing with broken promise.

But before you spend even a moment crying over spilled milk (or anti-aging cream, as the case may be), please read on. I think you'll be absolutely delighted to learn that your search for the Fountain of Youth has come to a very happy end. Through the program outlined in the pages of this book, you'll find the secret to young, beautiful skin that has led many an aspiring model to the covers of magazines!

Utilizing the extraordinarily effective approach to nutrition based on nucleic acid therapy and all-natural, yet customized, treatment products for daily care of the skin, you'll discover how you can literally turn back the face of time! Best of all, everything you need to effect such a dramatic change in your appearance is both inexpensive and readily available. As a matter of fact, you may have many of the necessary components in your own kitchen right now.

YOUR SKIN

Before getting into the specifics of this revolutionary plan, I'd like to equip you with a working knowledge of your skin, an accutely sensitive and highly reactive organ, susceptible to a wide variety of external and internal influences. This information will not only let you understand why my regime is so uniquely effective, but will also help you see why your prior attempts at self-improvement may have fallen somewhere short of expectation. *Here, then, is the inside story on your body's largest organ:*

The skin is made up of three layers: the *subcutaneous layer* (or fatty tissue); the *dermis* (which houses all of the blood vessels, nerves, sweat glands, and follicles), and the *epidermis* (which covers it all as the skin's outer layer).

Running through the dermis (and serving as its support system) is the *intercellular cement*, or connective tissue, consisting of collagen and elastin. This is what gives skin the resilience it needs to spring back to starting position after you flash a quick smile. But as you get older, it is quite common to find yourself still smiling long after the joke is through. This is because the intercellular cement starts to lose some of its grip with age until it eventually deteriorates, leaving the epidermis, which no longer has the support it needs to look firm, sagging into—you guessed it—a wrinkle.

This process can be either accelerated or retarded to quite a great extent. What happens depends, in large measure, on the degree to which one's skin is protected and properly cared for. To understand how this works, we have to explore each of the skin's major parts in a little more detail.

The Epidermis

The epidermis is built in several layers, each one with a different function. The *basal* (or lowest) layer is where the cells of the epidermis are born. These are plump, healthy cells that reproduce rapidly, gradually rising to the surface. As they move upward, however, they undergo many changes. One of the most important alterations is the increase in the amount of *keratin*, a cell-produced protein substance, within the cells. By the time the cells of the basal layer reach the top of the epidermis, they are no longer alive and are formed entirely of keratin.

Since keratin thrives on moisture to keep it pliable and healthy, it is essential that the skin be continually supplied with sufficient amounts of water, both internally and externally. If it is not, the keratin will crumble and the cells will become separated: This separation of cells is the cause of dry skin.

The skin's moisture (or hydration) level is dependent primarily on the *barrier* level. Made up of very thin cells, the barrier level is a membrane that controls the flow of water and oxygen into the skin as well as the evaporation and disposal of water and carbon dioxide out of the skin. This layer also contains a group of water-attracting compounds known as natural moisturizing factors (NMFs), including Sodium PCA. Sodium PCA (or NaPCA) is the most important natural moisturizer of the group because it determines the skin's ability to hold moisture. Old skin contains only one half of the NaPCA found in young skin. These compounds play a major role in maintaining a young, vibrant complexion. One reason older skin is usually drier is that the level of NMFs sharply decreases with age.

The epidermis' uppermost layer consists of old, dried cells that, having finished their "upward climb," tend to be parched and brittle. Composed mainly of keratin, these cells do not reproduce. Their primary function is to protect the layers lying directly beneath them: the exact area of the skin that cosmetic manufacturers refer to when they claim that this season's featured product penetrates "some twenty-three layers." In reality, none of these so-called treatments (intensive or otherwise) do any more than *temporarily* scratch the surface of the skin's uppermost and totally lifeless layer. If they were actually absorbed, as one would be led (or *mis*led) to believe, they would be classified a drug by the Food and Drug Administration and be sold only by prescription.

The Dermis

While most of the skin's problems are visible only on the epidermis, many are caused by troubles that originate in a deeper layer, the dermis. Made up of blood vessels, oil and sweat glands, the dermis is "glued" together by connective tissue that consists of collagen and elastin (neither of which have any lasting effect when applied topically).

It is the state of the skin's collagen that determines to what degree the complexion will wrinkle or scar. When the collagen fibers lose their flexibility because of age or are damaged by the sun or acne, the skin will wrinkle or sag because its underlying support structure is gone.

The Acid Mantle

A fluid that bathes the top layer of skin, the acid mantle is believed to act as a natural barrier of defense against infection, and is therefore of particular importance to the very oily or acneiform complexion (skin already predisposed to infection). The acid mantle is the natural acidity of the skin which helps to retard irritation or bacterial growth as well as maintain the skin's proper pH (acid/ alkaline balance).

HOW COSMETICS DO WHAT THEY DO

Now that you have a better understanding of the way in which the skin functions, it will be easier to see how you may have been hoodwinked by deceptive product claims in the past.

Before getting into specifics, I'd like to say that, by and large, the individual categories of products I'm about to discuss come about as close to delivering on their advertising claims as the star of the magic show comes to sawing the woman in half. In both cases, the end result is no more than an illusion and in the case of the former, it's a costly one at that, especially when their failure to perform is at the expense of your own self-esteem.

Here's how it's done. Since young skin reflects light much more efficiently than older skin does, cosmetic manufacturers try to re-create this phenomenon through a variety of artificial means. However, because the following "topical glazes" do not, in any way, change the structure of the skin, their very temporary effects are simply washed away with the nightly cleansing.

Line Preventors and Anti-Aging Complexes

This relatively new genre of gel-like liquid substances (Elizabeth Arden's Micro 2000 and Dior's Capture, for example) are touted as being unparalleled in their capacity to turn back the skin's biological clock, insuring your complexion a wrinkle-free tomorrow. What they actually accomplish is the very brief trapping of moisture in the uppermost epidermal layer. This temporarily "plumps out" minor lines and wrinkles, giving the skin a (short-lived) smoother, more even appearance. In addition, as the formula dries, the gel-like liquid leaves a coating that causes a slight tightening effect, momentarily disguising certain visible signs of age.

Texturizers

Also fairly new on the scene, this category of products (Luminique and Chanel's Blanc de Blanc are two) consists of ultra-light (practically white, sometimes iridescent) cremes or fluids. When patted gently over fine facial lines and scars, they are intended to reflect light from the depressed areas of the skin. Generally speaking, the improvement they bring is superficial, negligible, and very temporary.

Ampoules

Marketed with such descriptive phrases as "Intensive Care for the Skin" and produced by La Prairie, Charles of the Ritz, and many others, ampoules are easily recognizable because of the dosage-vial system in which they are usually packaged. Ostensibly, this is so the user can mix up a fresh batch each time she uses the product, a benefit whose validity is debatable.

It is most often recommended that ampoules be applied on a quarterly basis (that is, at the end of each season), at the rate of one vial every fourth day for four weeks. Thus there is some truth to the claim that they are intensive, although the same would hold true if *crude oil* were applied in a similar manner. The principle benefits of these most costly of treatment products is a marginal improvement in the tone of the skin, as well as a softened and therefore more light-refracting texture. Once again, however, both effects are *only temporary*.

STEP ONE ON YOUR ROAD TO BEAUTIFUL SKIN

Let's move on to the real matter at hand: the perfecting of the most important complexion in the room—*yours!*

The *single most important thing* you can do for the beauty of your skin is to establish your correct skintype. It is of vital (and *ongoing*) importance, and it's up to you to stay well informed. After all, can you really turn the responsibility of something that crucial over to the person behind the counter, someone who may very well be selling gloves that afternoon or children's clothing the next morning?

Like stunning shoes that are three sizes too small, no complexion can be shown off to its full advantage without a program of care that fits. Although you'll discover how to determine your particular type of skin in the chapter that follows, I want to emphasize the importance of always staying "on top" of it. Remember, a great many things can and do affect your skintype, causing it to change. If your regimen of care doesn't change along with it, the results can spell disaster. Take Julia M., for example.

A talented artist and sculptress, Julia's peaceful existence in tranquil Santa Fe, New Mexico, was turned upside down when a persuasive friend convinced her to move to New York City and join in the potentially lucrative co-ownership of a Madison Avenue art gallery.

Once in Manhattan, Julia became so consumed with the day-to-day business of running her new venture that she scarcely noticed the terrible effect her first summer in the city was having on her skin. With continual exposure to the chronic heat and exceptionally high levels of humidity, Julia's dry, blemish-free complexion was completely transformed, suddenly becoming oily and severely broken out (especially on her forehead, nose, and chin). When Labor Day arrived, her skin was in worse condition than it had ever been. She was in a state of total panic when a friend from the art world referred her to me.

After closely examining her face, I explained that her problems were, in large measure, a result of the change in climate. While the aridity of New Mexico may have allowed her to maintain a relatively trouble-free complexion, the city's intense humidity and its pollution were causing her skin to produce more oil. Since her regimen of care hadn't been adjusted accordingly, the additional oil was not being adequately removed. Left to accumulate, it had expanded the openings of her pores, causing the unwanted crop of blemishes to appear.

Continuing my probe, I asked Julia about her current diet. She sheepishly replied that, although good nutrition had always been a top priority for her before, the stress and sheer exhaustion she'd felt over the last few months had caused her to pay less attention to it. After confessing to subsisting mostly on junk food since she left Santa Fe, Julia readily acknowledged the obvious negative impact such neglect was having on her skin.

I outlined for Julia my program of daily care, as well as the nutritional and vitamin therapies that support it—all designed to normalize combination skin. She enthusiastically agreed to incorporate my suggestions into her life. Before she left, I prescribed an antibiotic to accelerate the healing of her acne.

By Christmastime, Julia's skin had indeed normalized, and all traces of acne had vanished. With the gallery a smashing success, she was once again able to relax and enjoy herself. At a holiday gathering, she said she even overheard two friends from college (neither of whom she'd seen in almost twenty years) say they thought she looked younger now than the last time they saw her (evidence that my anti-aging approach lives up to its name)!

These days, Julia divides her time between New York and Santa Fe. But by adapting her regimen to fit the locale, she's able to keep her complexion beautifully clear, regardless of the place she calls home. Let her example serve as reminder of the important role regular skintype "check-ups" (at least every six months) play in keeping your complexion at its vibrantly beautiful best.

WHY MY PROGRAM WORKS

Accomplished by means of a highly individualized regimen catering to the specific needs of each of the basic skintypes, my approach will guide you, step-by-step, through three thirty-day segments of care.

During the first month (when the plan's "core" is established), you will engage in a very detailed anti-aging diet and vitamin therapy regimen, along with a routine of customized daily skincare, complete with recipes for homemade products that *work*. You will also be armed with strategies for combating such common skin enemies as exposure to the elements and emotional stress. From the thirtieth to the sixtieth day, your program will be expanded to include treatments for such specialized problems as acne, sensitivity, and skin during pregnancy and menopause. The strategy builds to completion during the third thirty days, with the addition of in-depth advice for skincare under the sun as well as care of the body skin.

As an extra incentive, I've included lists of changes you can realistically expect to see in your complexion at the end of each thirty-day period. For example: a softening of surface facial wrinkles (such as those commonly found on the forehead, at the corners of the eyes, and between the nostrils and sides of the mouth) will be noticed after the first four to five weeks; all skin-types will begin to normalize (i.e. attain the correct balance between oily and dry) by the sixty-day mark; and the appearance of firmer, younger-looking skin on the back of the hands will be clearly evident at the end of ninety days. And while the plan is *initiated* over a period of three months, its benefits *will continue* for as long as its guidelines are followed.

The book's final portion is devoted to a comprehensive look at the latest in state-of-the-art cosmetic surgery procedures. There have been tremendous advances in recent years. Most people immediately think it's time to get a face lift when they see visible signs of aging on the face. But it's my opinion that far too many face lifts are being performed today. There are many simple cosmetic treatments which will take care of the majority of problems long before a face lift is necessary. Among them are fat injections and collagen treatments, methods for resurfacing the skin, filling in acne scars and wrinkles, and "tailoring" sagging flesh. All are explained here in detail. Also described are the ways in which the various procedures are performed (most, surprisingly, in the doctor's office), the follow-up care that is required, and what to realistically expect in the days and weeks following a cosmetic operation.

I'd like you to view *About Face* as your complete reference for the total care of your complexion, as truly an "owner's manual" for beautiful skin—and that, as we all know, is one thing that will never go out of style!

CHAPTER 2

Typing Your Skin

The first step on your road to a beautiful complexion is the determination of your skintype. This knowledge is *absolutely essential* to deriving maximum benefits from my plan. Countless women have come to me with severe skin problems, simply because they did not know their skintype and were sold the wrong product by the person behind the cosmetics counter. You can learn your correct skintype by performing the following, very brief self-examination:

Before washing your face in the morning (assuming it was clean when you went to bed), take a piece of tissue paper and press it lightly over your facial skin surface. Hold the tissue paper in place for approximately thirty seconds, then gently remove it. Examine the paper. If it's clean, your skin probably falls into the category of "dry." A T imprint indicates a "combination" complexion. And if you've left your mask, you most likely have an "oily" skin. This test is valid for all skins, regardless of race or nationality.

To verify your results, compare the characteristics of your own skin with those listed under the three skintypes below. This review should reinforce your findings and put you on the right track of care for your particular complexion.

Oily Skin (see pages 15 to 59)

❍ Pores are visibly enlarged.
❍ Thick- or rough-textured.
❍ Shiny, greasy feel; hard to keep makeup in place.
❍ Usually troubled by some form of acne.
❍ Generally youthful in appearance; no signs of premature aging.

Combination Skin (see pages 61 to 104)

❍ Pores visible on nose and sometimes on chin
❍ Slightly coarse in texture.
❍ Appears oily in T-zone (forehead, nose, and chin); dry around eyes, cheeks, and neck.
❍ Whiteheads and blackheads are often apparent.
❍ Nose and chin begin to shine two to three hours after makeup is applied.

Dry Skin (see pages 105 to 147)

❍ Very fine pores.
❍ Texture is "flat" or dull to the touch.
❍ Shows early signs of aging (premature wrinkles and lines).
❍ Tends to itch, flake, and become easily chapped.
❍ Frequently has patches of blotchiness, brown spots, or both.

A variety of factors—from diet to climate to emotions to aging—can cause skintypes to change. Therefore, it is essential that you give yourself periodic "rechecks," especially if you feel your skincare regimen isn't performing up to par. Also, if your skin is very easily irritated and often blotchy in appearance, it's probably *sensitive* as well as dry, combination, or oily.

Once you've established your skintype, you're ready to embark on the treatment route that corresponds to it. Within the pages indicated above, you will find your definitive, all-in-one guide to perfect skin in ninety days, and for *the rest of your life* as well!

My Ninety-Day [   ] Plan for Oily Skin

PART I

Although an oily complexion is usually the most problematic early in life, it tends to age far more gracefully than any other type of skin, because of its inherent extra thickness.

Through careful adherence to my lifestyle plan, however, those with oily skin no longer have to wait for their "twilight" years to start enjoying a beautiful complexion. It can be theirs *anytime*, regardless of age. The components of my program work to regulate the skin's excess production of oil and, in so doing, not only normalize it but also greatly reduce any occurrence of acne. The end result: a very attractive complexion.

When Catherine G. first came to see me, she was in a state of complete despair over the condition of her skin. Although at age 26 she was a very successful model and cover girl, recent outbreaks of eraser-sized blemishes around her mouth and chin were preventing her from pursuing further work as a face model, her area of specialization. The makeup artists who strove to hide her imperfections from the camera's eye were at the bottom of their bags of concealment tricks and suggested she seek professional help.

I began by assuring her that the situation was not nearly as hopeless as she perceived it to be and that within no time I would have her back to her clear-complected self. I explained that she was suffering from a relatively newly identified form of acne known as perioral dermatitis. Afflicting mostly young women (especially those prone to oily skin), the condition appears to be primed by the use of fluoride toothpastes and to be exacerbated by greasy cover-up cremes and cosmetics. A vicious cycle of perpetual redness and irritation to the lower portion of the face is created.

I recommended she start by substituting her regular toothpaste (containing fluoride) with one made by combining five parts baking soda with one part hydrogen peroxide (an excellent tooth whitener). Further, I suggested she follow my program for the daily care of oily skin (limiting herself to the use of water-based makeups), as well as my anti-aging nutritional and vitamin therapy plans. Finally, to bring her problem under control in the fastest possible time, I prescribed an antibiotic to accelerate healing of her lesions.

Today, Catherine works exclusively as a face model and is much in demand. She has, in fact, recently signed with one of the major cosmetic companies as their representative. Her complexion is flawless, and she's filled with renewed hope for a long and prosperous career. Incidentally, she's discovered an additional benefit to following my anti-aging nutritional plan—she no longer has to watch her weight!

During our initial consultation, Jessica M. told me she was completely baffled by the fact that her once controllable oily skin had suddenly blossomed into a full-blown case of acne. A world-class tennis pro and avid health enthusiast, she had lately even incorporated long-distance running and megadoses of vitamins (including vitamin-B12 injections) into her personal fitness regime. It therefore seemed especially ironic to her that such problems should arise.

I agreed that she had every right to feel confused but explained that, strangely enough, her problems probably stemmed from too much of a good thing. Certain vitamins—especially shots of B12 and massive doses of vitamin E—can bring on a condition (particularly in the oily-skinned individual) known as vitamin acne. Her course of treatment, therefore, began by discontinuing the B12 injections entirely and switching, instead, to a good B-complex tablet (containing at least 150 mg. of both vitamins B2 and B6, two oil controllers). To further personalize her anti-aging nutritional and vitamin therapy plans, I reduced her vitamin E intake to 100 I.V.s per day and, using her skin's reaction as a guide, very gradually increased the dosage to a daily maximum, in her case, of 400 I.V.s.

Of additional concern to Jessica was an everpresent strip of whiteheads around her hairline, which I informed her was caused by the sweatband she wore over the area while running and playing tennis. These bands, by the way, do much more trapping than absorbing of perspiration and are frequently the culprit when it comes to such localized irritation. Keeping one's hair clean and off the face *entirely* is the best way to prevent additional oil from seeping onto the skin. I also suggested she carry a few medicated pads (such as Noxzema Clear-Ups) with her to absorb excess oil during and immediately following her workouts. Through careful attention to every recommended detail, Jessica regained control of her complexion in record time. She reports that her stamina and energy levels have never been higher and that she's now able to enjoy all the benefits her very healthy lifestyle affords her.

These are just two of the countless number of oily-skinned patients whose complexions (and often lives) have been dramatically improved after embarking upon my plan of specialized care. And from this moment on, you too can begin to derive these same benefits. All of the information you need to get started is contained in the pages to follow, so let's not delay. After all, there's a whole new you just waiting to be discovered!

My Ninety-Day Plan for Oily Skin

The First Thirty Days: De-aging the Skin

DAILY CARE

Your personal care, every day, is the most important element in maintaining beautiful, young-looking skin; without a meticulously cared-for complexion, one can never hope to fulfill one's true beauty potential. With this in mind, I've developed the following "natural alternatives" to more traditional treatment products. Created especially for use on oily skin, the formulas are all very easy to prepare, inexpensive, and extremely effective. Once you've tried them and seen for yourself the difference they can make, I'm certain you'll never use another thing on your face.

Here is your program of daily care:

Morning

STEP 1: CLEANSING. Apply 2 or 3 tablespoons of plain natural yogurt (very soothing) to damp skin and massage well over face and throat area. Follow with 20 splashes of tepid water to insure that no residue remains on the skin.

STEP 2: TONING. After cleansing, stir 1 teaspoon of apple cider vinegar into an 8-ounce glass of water (more if skin is very sensitive). Apply to face and throat with pads of cotton in an upward sweeping motion. Besides being a very efficient toner, this preparation will restore the acid balance, or normal pH, to skin. *To soothe erupted skin*, try toning with the following: 2 ounces of grapefruit juice mixed with 2 ounces of vodka and 3 ounces of mineral water. The vitamins A and C contained in the grapefruit juice will help to dry and heal the blemishes, while the vodka will aid in tightening the pores. This mixture may be stored in a small bottle or jar and kept refrigerated for a week.

STEP 3: NOURISHING. While skin is still damp, lock in moisture by applying one of the three nourishing suggestions that follow, *only* to dry areas, such as around the eyes.

Either: A thin layer of margarine (the kind sold in health food stores) that contains no artificial flavorings, colorings, or preservatives. (Amazingly, when topically applied, the margarine sinks right into skin, leaving no greasy residue.)

Or: A light application of mayonnaise. To insure its quality, try making it yourself, using the following recipe:

> To 1 slightly beaten egg yolk, add a cup of olive oil, 1 teaspoon at a time. When the mixture starts to thicken, whisk in a teaspoon of fresh lemon juice, and voilà—the "makings" of smooth skin! Mayonnaise can be stored in a similar manner as the toner, but make a fresh batch every four or five days. Also, be sure to stir before each use.

Or: If mayonnaise or margarine don't appeal to you, a light application of olive or any cold-pressed oil is also good.

Evening

STEP 1: MAKEUP REMOVAL. Any thin, natural, cold-pressed oil may be used for this purpose, with avocado, olive, and safflower oils all registering as popular choices. Simply massage oil lightly over the face and throat, removing it with pads of damp cotton. Repeat until the last traces of oil and makeup have disappeared. By the way, these oils penetrate only the top layers of skin, where the protection and conditioning they provide are very much needed. When used in this manner, they will not cause the skin to break out.

STEP 2: CLEANSING. Same as in the morning.

STEP 3: EXFOLIATING. Necessary for removing the dead cell accumulation that naturally occurs on all types of skin, this procedure is particularly beneficial to the oily-skinned individual when it is performed on a daily basis. Several readily available products may be used for exfoliating, including sea salt, yellow cornmeal, and white sugar. The latter also benefits skin by having a slightly antibacterial effect.

To make a paste, start by adding a teaspoon of water to a small amount of any one of the three ingredients, gradually increasing the moisture content until a desired consistency is reached. Then, *gently* massage the mixture over the entire face and throat area with tips of fingers to loosen debris from the surface of pores. Finish by rinsing well with warm water, followed by a cool splash. (*Please note*: This procedure should not be performed on areas of the face where active acne is present.)

STEP 4: TONING. Same as in the morning.

STEP 5: NOURISHING. Same as in the morning.

Extra Help

MASKS. To enhance the effects of any mask, gently steam your face before applying. Simply toss a few bags of chamomile tea into a pot of boiling water, remove from stove, and, draping a towel over your head in a tentlike fashion, capture the steam.

Masks should be made fresh for each use.

The masks you can prepare yourself are nearly as varied as those you can buy. Always apply them to clean skin, and try to use a mask once or twice a week. Here are a few of the most effective masks I've discovered:

> **For clarifying oily skin.** Combine 1 egg white with the juice of ½ freshly squeezed lemon and 1 tablespoon of plain yogurt. Apply to clean face and remove with warm water after mask has been allowed to dry for 20 minutes.

> **For a super peeling.** Combine 1 tablespoon of almonds (finely ground in blender) with the same amount of honey

and 1 egg white. Allow to dry on face for 15 to 20 minutes. Remove by massaging with warm water in a rotating motion over skin. Rinse well.

For a satiny smooth texture and radiant glow. Mix 2 tablespoons of brewer's yeast powder with 1 tablespoon of aloe vera juice and 1 egg white. Stir into a thick paste and allow to remain on face for 30 minutes before removing with warm water. This mask will also help to heal blemishes and soothe irritated skin.

TOPICAL TREATMENTS AND WHY THEY WORK SO WELL

Apple cider vinegar. Restores skin to proper pH (acid/alkaline) balance.

Lemon. Rich in vitamin C, potassium, and iron, it gives tone to the skin and acts as a mild bleach.

Nail-polish remover. When applied with cotton-tipped swab to *individual blemishes only*, the acetone it contains rapidly dries the lesions, thus accelerating the healing process.

Oatmeal or Wheatena. Gently exfoliates and deep-cleanses the skin. It also soothes irritations.

Vodka. As a very pure form of alcohol, it is a very effective astringent for tightening pores.

White sugar. An extremely efficient skin exfoliant, with the added advantage of having a slightly antibacterial effect on the complexion.

Yogurt. Cleanses and soothes the skin; reduces visible signs of irritation.

Milk of magnesia. Has a very healing effect on acne. Since it is slightly drying to the skin, its usage should be confined to individual lesions only.

For a calming effect. Mix 1 tablespoon of wheat germ with 1 tablespoon of yogurt. Apply to skin, and allow to remain for 15 minutes before removing with tepid water. This mask is especially good for an irritated complexion.

For healing a blemished complexion. Soak 1 slice of white bread and 1 cube of yeast in ¼ cup of milk and allow to stand until a paste forms. Apply to skin, and leave on for 30 minutes. Remove with warm water.

For reducing inflammation. For inflamed and blemished skin, apply yogurt lightly over entire face and leave for 30 minutes. Remove with a damp white baby's washcloth. (Use a fresh one each time.) Or simply remove with warm water from sink or shower. Follow removal with a cool splash.

TO HYDRATE THE SKIN. Skin is dehydrated if it appears blotchy as well as dry. Dehydrated skin should respond quickly to extra moisture (water, not oil).

Oily skin can become dehydrated just as easily as any other type, as it's the *water* content of skin that determines its level of moisture and *not* the oil. For intense skin hydration, such as is needed after overexposure to the elements, I've found the following treatment unbeatable:

Apply predigested liquid protein with soluble collagen (the kind once used, rather dangerously, for dieting and still available at most health food stores) evenly over face and neck. (A wooden tongue depressor—available at most drug stores—may be used for this purpose.) Allow to dry and remain on skin for 1 or 2 hours, lightly spritzing the area with water at 15 to 20-minute intervals. Rinse well after allotted time has passed. The hydrating effect this has on skin seems to last for several days following application.

TO DRY ACNE LESIONS. Apply nail-polish remover directly onto the blemish with a cotton-tipped swab. The acetone in the formula will aid in drying up the lesion. (*One note*: As some nail-polish removers are now acetone-free, be sure to check for this ingredient before purchasing for this purpose.)

Milk of magnesia applied in the same manner will produce a similar effect; its less-harsh formula makes it a wiser choice for those with more sensitive skin.

TO REDUCE PUFFINESS AROUND EYES. *Either*: Obtain 2 slices from inside of potato and place over closed eyes. Rest in this position for 15 minutes prior to applying makeup.

Or: Use tea bags that have been dipped in hot water and then chilled. Apply in the same manner. Incidentally, the cheaper brands of tea are usually highest in tannic acid, the ingredient that produces the desired effect.

Or: Sleeping on two or three pillows at night.

TO FADE RED SPOTS ON SKIN. Combine 1 tablespoon each of freshly squeezed lemon juice and salt. Using a cotton-tipped swab, place mixture directly on reddened areas. After 10 minutes, rinse well.

NUTRITION AND VITAMIN THERAPY

Building Strength from Within

Have you ever heard anyone ask, ''Is it surgery or sardines?'' as they pondered the reason for someone's particularly young, attractive appearance? While the answer to that query could be a combination of the two, you may not be aware of the significant role the lowly sardine can play in maintaining beautiful skin.

On the anti-aging nutritional team, the sardine could easily be voted most valuable player, for this humble fish has the profound distinction of being the only food to double its already high content of RNA (ribonucleic acid) and DNA (deoxyribonucleic acid) while in the can.

RNA and DNA are the ''stuff cells are made of.'' And cells—by the millions—are the things that make up our bodies, each with a lifespan of approximately two years. Before the cell dies, it reproduces itself on orders given by a commander-in-chief (DNA) and carried out by a messenger (RNA). In theory, therefore, we should look the same today as we did ten or fifteen years ago. But unfortunately, as with most theories, this one has holes in it.

Because of a variety of external factors beyond our control, the cell goes through some deterioration with each successive reproduction, causing an alteration in its shape. The further away it moves from its original blueprint, the more visibly we show signs of aging.

Interestingly and very encouragingly, however, the matter is not entirely out of our hands. Work pioneered by the late Benjamin Frank, M.D. demonstrated that if we keep our bodies well supplied with external sources of the nucleic acids (like sardines), we can rejuvenate the cells to the point where the aging process is drastically retarded or even reversed. In addition, we will be contributing to an overall improvement in appearance as well as to a general sense of well-being. And therein lies the basis for my anti-aging nutritional plan, which will, if carefully followed, change much more than simply the way you eat.

So if you're ready to start feeling stronger, thinking more clearly, aging more slowly, and looking much, much better, I invite you to proceed to the specifics of the plan.

My Anti-aging Nutritional Plan*

Four days per week, a 3- or 4-ounce can of sardines must be eaten. Since you do not need the excess oil in your diet, opt for the water-packed variety.

Three other days per week, have one of the following: a serving of salmon, tuna, sole, bluefish, scrod, or monkfish. (Avoid crustaceans.)

Once or twice a week, have a serving of liver (chicken liver is best).

Have 2 or 3 eggs each week if your cholesterol level is not elevated. (If there is a question, check with your doctor.)

Everyday include 1 serving of fresh pineapple or papaya, in addition to 1 serving of any other fresh fruit.

Twice a week, have a serving of lentils, peas, lima beans, or soybeans.

Each day, have a salad prepared with some or all of the following ingredients: lettuce, mushrooms, asparagus, radishes, celery, beets, carrots, and broccoli. No spinach or onions.

*If you are currently under a physician's care, check with your doctor before embarking on this or any other specialized nutritional program.

Have 1 tablespoon each of bran, wheat germ, brewer's yeast, and lecithin granules daily.

Two or three times per week, have a serving of oatmeal or Wheatena.

Include in your daily beverage intake all of the following: 1 glass of fruit or vegetable juice, 1 glass of skimmed milk (unless cystic acne is a problem), and 6 to 8 glasses (8 oz.) of pure water (preferably bottled).

Have oat bran muffins for breakfast frequently. It lowers cholesterol and is great for fiber.

Finally enjoy this daily "beauty cocktail": Mix 3 tablespoons liquid acidophilus (found in health food stores and containing friendly bacteria) and 1 tablespoon lactose (also found in health food stores) into an 8-ounce glass of water, and drink to good health . . . yours! The good bacteria in this cocktail will help destroy and eliminate toxins from the body.

If you stick strictly to this diet—with no additions—you'll lose weight. If weight is not a problem for you, the aforementioned foods may be incorporated into your regular diet, provided it does not include any of the following foods, which must be *avoided*. If this proves to be difficult, certainly try to *minimize* them in your diet.

Anything containing white flour or sugar; for sweetening, small amounts of honey or blackstrap molasses make healthy alternatives.

Alcoholic beverages; try a sparkling water like Perrier or Pellegrino and lemon or lime instead.

Red meat; dark poultry meat is all right.

Salt; garlic can be used in many instances as a substitute.

Fats; cold-pressed oils, such as safflower, are permitted in moderation.

Products containing caffeine; herbal teas are fine.

Bringing on the Reinforcements

Each day, include the following vitamin and mineral supplements in your diet:

One high-potency multivitamin containing chelated minerals after breakfast. (''Chelated'' is your key to no stomach upset from certain supplements. Look for it on labels.)

One RNA/DNA tablet (125 mg.) daily after lunch. (Not to exceed daily intake of 150 mg—including multivitamin.)

Two high-potency B-complex vitamin tablets, one after breakfast and one after lunch. (Not to exceed total daily intake—including multivitamins—of 100 mg. each of: Vit. B-1, Vit. B-2, Vit. B-6, and Vit. D, and 100 mcg. of Vit. B-12, 400 mcg. of folic acid, and 300 mcg. of Biotin.) B-complex vitamins are especially important for women taking birth control pills.

Two vitamin C tablets with bioflavinoids (500 mg. each), each after eating. (Not to exceed total daily intake including multivitamin—of 1,000 mg.) Higher dose may cause stomach upset.

Vitamin E (800 I.U.s, dry form), once a day after breakfast. (Not to exceed total daily intake including multivitamins of 800 I.U.s)

Selenium (50 mcg.) once a day, taken in conjunction with vitamin E. (Not to exceed intake of 100 mcg.—including multivitamin.)

Vitamin A (10,000 I.U.s) daily after lunch. (Not to exceed total daily intake—including multivitamin—of 20,000 I.U.s)

Chelated zinc (50 mg.) daily after breakfast. (Not to exceed intake of 100 mg.—including multivitamin—each day.)

Cysteine, an amino acid (500 mg.), midafternoon with

a glass of either orange or grapefruit juice. (Not to exceed intake of 500 mg. daily—including multivitamin.)

If this seems like a lot to swallow, imagine what a bitter pill it would be to discover, too late, that many of your blemishes, lines, and wrinkles were preventable.

Putting the Plan into Action for You

What follows is an outline of a typical day on my anti-aging nutritional plan.

BREAKFAST.

High-energy shake made with:

> 8 ounces skim milk
> ½ cup fresh raspberries
> 1 tablespoon each, brewer's yeast and lecithin granules
> Honey, to taste
> 2–3 ice cubes (for thickness)
>
> Mix on high speed in blender until frothy.

Bowl of cooked oatmeal sprinkled with 1 tablespoon each of bran and wheat germ.

Herbal tea

After breakfast, the following supplements:

> 1 high-potency multivitamin/multimineral
> 1 vitamin B-complex tablet
> 500 mg. vitamin C with bioflavinoids
> 800 I.U.s vitamin E (dry form)
> 100 mcg. selenium
> 50 mg. chelated zinc

SUGGESTED FOODS AND HOW THEY BENEFIT YOUR SYSTEM

Sardines. Highest single source of nucleic acids (RNA/DNA). The only food to double such content while in the can.

Oatmeal or Wheatena. Also a good source of RNA/DNA, as well as natural fiber. When paired with bran, has been shown to be effective in reducing levels of cholesterol.

Papaya. Contains valuable digestive properties as well as valuable nutrients.

Lentils. Excellent alternate source of protein; also rich in nucleic acid.

Lecithin. Used in the making of chocolate to keep it from hardening before its time; has a similar effect on one's arteries. Also, an important moisture-binding agent.

Yogurt. Furnishes useful bacteria that keep the intestines clean by countering toxic substances.

The reason for one firm "no no"—alcohol. Especially when taken with meals, it tends to raise levels of uric acid, the very thing the diet strives to prevent by emphasizing fluids.

LUNCH.

Platter of hors d'oevres that includes:

3–4 ounces (water-packed) sardines
Beet slices
Celery and asparagus stalks
Raw broccoli
1–2 tablespoons cooked lentils
1–2 tablespoons freshly squeezed lemon juice sprinkled on top

Serving of fresh pineapple

Perrier and lime

After lunch, these supplements:

125 mg. RNA/DNA tablet
10,000 I.U.s vitamin A
1 vitamin B-complex tablet

MIDAFTERNOON.

500 mg. cysteine with 4 ounces of grapefruit juice

DINNER.

Lettuce and tomato salad

Broiled chicken livers

Steamed peas and carrots

Dish of fresh strawberries

Herbal tea

After dinner, this supplement:

500 mg. vitamin C with bioflavinoids

If weight is not a problem for you, the aforementioned meals may be augmented as you wish, excluding, of course, the foods listed on the "to be avoided" roster.

Last, but not least, be creative! And remember to view each and every dining experience as the wonderfully rejuvenating treat for your skin that it is.

Sardine "Surprises"

Sardines are an amazingly versatile (not to mention incredibly healthy) food that should be eaten often. Here are a few innovative ways to maximize their appeal:

Peppers Stuffed with Sardines

2 large green peppers
3½ oz. can sardines (water packed), chopped
1 cup cooked rice
1½ medium-sized onion, minced
½ cup tomato sauce
1 egg
Salt and pepper

With a paring knife, cut a circle around the stem of each pepper. Pull out the stems, and, with a fork or teaspoon, scrape away as many of the seeds from the hollow as you can. Rinse them out with cold water.

Mix the sardines with the rice, the onion, and the tomato sauce. Beat the egg and add this along with approximately ½ teaspoon of salt and a dash of pepper.

Put this mixture into the hollow peppers, and bake for about 20 minutes at 350° F.

Sardines with Gouda Cheese

This makes a superb easy-to-cook main dish for two.

    2 3½ oz. cans sardines
    1 pound spinach
    1½ cup skimmed milk
    3 tablespoons corn oil margarine
    3 tablespoons flour
    2 teaspoons Worcestershire sauce
    ¾ cup crumbled Gouda cheese

Drain the sardines into a large frying pan, and set the sardines aside.

Wash the spinach and tear it into bite-sized pieces. Heat the sardine oil and pile spinach onto it. Cover and cook over low heat for 5 minutes, until the margarine melts.

While the spinach is cooking put 1 cup of the skimmed milk into a saucepan with the margarine. Heat over very low heat until the margarine melts.

Mix the flour into the rest of the skimmed milk, and pour the mixture slowly into the heating milk while stirring. Add the Worcestershire sauce, and all but 3 tablespoons of the cheese. Continue stirring until cheese melts, making sure the mixture does not boil.

Put the cooked spinach into a greased baking dish. Then, place the sardines on top of the spinach and the cheese sauce on top of everything. Sprinkle the rest of the cheese on this, and bake at 400° F until the cheese melts (about 10 minutes).

A Canapé

Very lightly toast 2 slices of white bread. Cut each slice into 4 pieces. Mash 3½ ounces of sardines with a fork and spread over the bread pieces. Top with a few shavings of Swiss cheese and bake at 350°, until the cheese melts.

COMBATING THE SABOTEURS OF YOUNG SKIN

The time bandits that fall into this category have been guilty of bringing on an "early frost" in more cases than I'd care to remember, so let's examine the ways in which each of them contribute to the skin's demise and, more importantly, what can be done to minimize the damage.

For starters, you have an extremely powerful ally in your running battle with time, running right out of your kitchen and bathroom faucets! That's right, good old H_2O can be your single best defense when it comes to beating the clock, so be sure to take full advantage. Since, however, one can never be sure of the quality of tap water, it's best to either install a charcoal filter or drink the bottled variety.

The following are some of water's many and varied uses, which are especially important for oily skin. I strongly suggest you immediately incorporate each of them into your daily life:

> Increase your consumption of the liquid by having at least 1 quart each day. This will aid in the removal of toxins from your system, which in turn will prevent them from having a negative impact on your skin (especially important for clearing a blemished complexion). Keep a pitcher of chilled water in the refrigerator at all times. For a refreshing and slightly tangy change of pace, try adding a few slices of fresh lemon to the container before storing.

> If you haven't done so already, purchase a humidifier and keep it going in your bedroom while you sleep.* It's a small investment that will pay big dividends in moisture restored to your skin. (Be sure to change the water daily.)

> When washing your face, always rinse with twenty splashes of tepid water. Rehydrate often throughout the day by "spritzing" the area with one of the mineral waters (Evian, for example) sold in an aerosol can. This

---

*Be sure to change your bed linens (especially pillow cases) often, to insure that you don't reexpose your face to the same "pregreased" surface every night.

is especially important when traveling by air, as the pressurized cabins are extremely drying to skin. For the same reason, make your cocktails Perrier or another bottled water instead of alcohol.

Sun

Because of the overwhelmingly negative impact the sun has on skin, I've devoted an entire section ("Sun specifics" in "The Third Thirty Days: Completing the Plan,") for your enlightenment. Precautions should be taken at all times—no matter what the weather. But if you're planning a vacation to the tropics, where intense sun exposure is imminent, extra precautions should be taken immediately.

Exposure

When it comes to the aging effects of the elements (wind, heat, cold), total avoidance is your best defense, even though your oily and thus thicker skin does "weather the storm" better than other types. Unfortunately, from the day you leave the hospital in your mother's arms, this is a virtually impossible task, so the next best thing is to always take the proper precautions. Be sure to apply sun screen with an SPF of at least 15 to your face, neck, and backs of the hands each morning (alone or under make-up); wear sunglasses all year round whenever you're exposed to the sun, regardless of the temperature; wear protective clothing (i.e. heat reflecting in the summer and insulated in the winter, including hats and gloves).

When I speak of "the elements," you probably think this refers only to the ones we're exposed to out of doors. On the contrary, the seasonal accommodations we make indoors (central heating and air conditioning) are every bit as detrimental to the health of your skin as their fresh-air counterparts. (Remember, it's water, not oil, that keeps skin moist.) Therefore, environmental protection on both fronts is definitely in order. Don't forget the humidifier. This is especially important in winter. Also, keep plants around. They're good for the skin.

Be sure your skincare routine changes whenever your wardrobe does. Winter's cold and gusty winds are far more drying to skin than summer's heat and humidity, so be certain to cleanse, tone, and moisturize accordingly.

Facial Stress

Squinting, sneering, scowling, pursing the lips, knitting the brow—all are common, everyday habits that happen to be major contributing factors to a condition known as facial stress: the self-inflicted damage done to facial muscles through chronic grimacing and general fatigue.

Although these reflexes are in some cases deeply ingrained in the mannerisms of an individual, for most people an awareness of their existence is usually all it takes to arrest the problem.

A patient once came to see me requesting collagen injections in the furrows of her brow. After noting the wrinkle-free appearance of the rest of her face, I advised that she might unconsciously be causing or aggravating the lines. To verify this fact, I suggested that she place a mirror on her desk at work and one near her telephone at home.

By setting up a ''wrinkle watch'' in this manner, she became aware that she was fervently knitting her brow during every telephone conversation. Once the collagen injections had corrected the problem, I suggested she might avoid a recurrence by placing small strips of hair-setting tape over the susceptible areas while at home. The slight tightening effect this produced at every twist and turn served as a more than sufficient deterrent whenever her face decided to ''go into motion.''

The same technique can be applied to any area of the face that is noticeably more lined than the rest. By closely observing the bad habits you probably didn't even realize you had, you can usually put a stop to them and, hence, the damage that results.

Now that you know how to stop these facial distortions ''in their tracks'' (or hopefully before they've left any permanent ones on your face), here are some other ways they get their start:

> Smoking is a double offender. Inhaling entails the pursing of the lips, while exhaling causes the eyes to squint (a reaction of self-defense to prevent the smoke from entering). In addition, smoking depletes the body's supply of Vitamin C, vital for its production of collagen.

Another frequent cause of squinting is poor vision. To avoid this problem, see your ophthalmologist regularly, and keep your prescription for *corrective lenses* up to date.

Making a concerted effort to get all the sleep you need (for most this means the standard eight hours per night) can be a great beauty boon, as a lack of sleep really does "show on your face" and aggravate the oiliness in your complexion, as well. Skin cells repair and rejuvenate themselves during periods of slumber, so opt for nine hours whenever possible.

Try training yourself to sleep on your back (or at least start the night out in that position). It just might help put an end to the formation of lines and wrinkles that are a result of your face pressing against the pillow night after night. (Satin-cased pillows are best, by the way.)

The Use and Abuse of Alcohol

In addition to dehydrating the system and depleting the body's supply of the B vitamins, long-term consumption of alcohol can lead to dilation of the blood vessels. Eventually this can result in a condition known as rosacea, which gives the nose a red, blotchy, bulbous appearance. And let's face it, no matter how popular a nostalgia craze becomes, you might long for Cleopatra's eyes and adore Mona Lisa's smile, but one look no one will ever want to imitate is that of W. C. Fields's nose (the most famous case of rosacea)! If you're not already "on the wagon," for your skin's sake, please climb aboard.

Emotional Stress

It flushes with embarrassment and rage, and it blanches with fear. There's no doubt about it, your skin truly is your body's emotional barometer.

If you have any doubt about just how aging chronic stress can be, compare two photographs of almost any official elected to high public office: one taken upon entering, the other on leaving the job. Such an image is worth more than a thousand words of warning. I treat many of these individuals, and, as a group, they challenge my skills for holding time at bay more than any other.

Since, however, stress is a fact of life that can never be completely eliminated, we must find a way (anything from self-hypnosis to psychotherapy) of handling it. The important thing is to discover a relaxation technique that works for you and to practice it regularly.

Lack of Exercise

Besides being a great source of stress relief (especially the aerobic variety), exercise flushes impurities out of the system through perspiration, improves circulation by carrying increased oxygen to cells, and firms and tones the muscles. It should therefore be apparent to even the greatest skeptic that exercise plays a vital role in postponing the visible signs of aging. Exercise is the body's fountain of youth.

If you're not currently engaged in a regular sport—whether it be walking, jogging, swimming, or bicycling—find an activity you enjoy, start slowly, and build up the pace. Three times a week for at least a half hour is essential for cardio-pulmonary function as well as for terrific skin. The vast improvement in the way you look and feel will serve as more than sufficient incentive for continuing.

In addition, you can reverse the pull of gravity, to a certain extent, by standing on your head or lying on a slantboard with your feet elevated for ten minutes each day. (Any 6- to 8-foot-long plank of wood—at least 10 inches wide—can be used.) Along with increasing the flow of blood to the dermis (creating a glow in the complexion), this action is an excellent energizer. (*A word of warning*: This position can cause extra pressure on the eyes. For those who are predisposed to conditions such as glaucoma, it could create or aggravate a problem. It is therefore best to check with your doctor before beginning).

Rapid and Frequent Changes in Weight

If you abuse your body by subjecting it to the "yo-yo" dieting syndrome, you are doing your skin more of a disservice than if you remained consistently overweight. The skin's elasticity is by no means "snap-proof," and if the body's supply of fat is constantly being depleted and restored, its resiliency simply wears out. Left with improper support, the irreversibly stretched skin can be likened to a tent at the end of camping season, once you've collapsed the pole; the canvas is left to drape loosely over whatever remains.

Early in my career, I treated one such individual. Anna P. first came to see me to discuss ways in which her sagging facial skin (the result of a 100-pound weight loss) could be tightened. Although, as I suspected, it was the same 100 pounds she had gained and lost countless times before, she assured me that this time the loss was permanent. Besides having maintained her current weight for close to four years, she said she now held an executive position with the weight-loss organization that had inspired her success and was under constant pressure there to stay thin. She felt the current state of her skin made her look a good twenty years older than she really was, and I agreed.

Several weeks following that first visit, Anna underwent a face lift. She was so pleased with the results of the cosmetic surgery that she went on to have a tummy tuck as well as liposuction in those few areas that exercise just wouldn't budge.

Today Anna looks like the daughter of the woman who originally came to see me. And although her life is now rich and rewarding in every way, she deeply regrets having spent the time and trouble she could have saved had she not subjected her body to such early abuse.

Heredity

It's been said that you can choose your friends but not your relatives. And since genetic composition is the single most determining factor when it comes to assessing the rate at which your skin will age, one look at your family can either make your hopes for maintaining a youthful complexion soar or send them plummeting into the depths of despair.

If your senior-citizen parents are constantly being mistaken for your second-grader's mom and dad, rejoice! You've probably inherited a wonderful set of genes. If, on the other hand, your folks looked like senior citizens even when *you* were in the second grade, don't fret, for all is not lost. Your "aging destiny" is by no means cast in iron. Rather, it happens to be quite flexible and capable of change.

By carefully nurturing and protecting the support structure of your body's largest organ, you will be able to hold back the signs of time in your skin for years to come and, in so doing, will change the course of (your family's aging) history!

CHANGES TO EXPECT AFTER THIRTY DAYS

Oily skin will become less so; signs of acne will start to diminish.

Surface facial wrinkles (such as those that commonly appear on the forehead, at the corners of eyes, and between the nostrils and the sides of the mouth) will soften.

Feelings of lethargy will subside, replaced by a resurgence of energy.

Symptoms of insomnia will start to disappear; a general sense of well-being will be experienced.

The Second Thirty Days: Treating Special Problems

ACNE

This four-letter word spells *trouble,* a fact to which its millions of hapless victims can unequivocally attest. Luckily, help has finally arrived! Through the pages of this chapter, you'll become privy to all of the information you'll need to put your problems with acne well behind you, once and for all.

My strategic defense plan begins with a little background material on your opponent, the world's most prevalent skin disease, and goes on to tell you what changes in lifestyle will do to improve your complexion, as well as what can be done about the problem *right now.*

The ''Family'' of Acne Lesions

Definitely not the sort to which you'd willingly extend an invitation, the members of this clan are the kind that tend to show up uninvited. Before we proceed any further, I'd like to make you aware of the wide variety of forms this most unwelcome intruder can take.

How Acne Begins

The skin is made up of three layers: the subcutaneous layer (or fatty tissue); the dermis (which houses the blood vessels, nerves, sweat glands, and follicles); and the epidermis (which covers the dermis and serves as the skin's "overcoat"). Running through the dermis is the connective tissue that, as its name implies, is the supporting structure of the dermis.

While the sweat glands have a direct opening to the surface of the skin, the oil (or sebaceous) glands are not quite as fortunate. The oil (or sebum) produced in these glands must find its way to the skin's surface via a follicle or pore, some of which contain hair. This is where the trouble can get its start. If the cells that line these follicles stick together instead of sloughing off (as they do under normal conditions), acne begins, and all forms of acne initiate in the very same manner. Now for a closer look:

MICROCOMEDO. This earliest form of acne plug is not visible to the naked eye. Nonetheless, microcomedones are insidious and can (and often do) lead to more serious things.

CLOSED COMEDO. This more advanced stage of the microcomedo is also called a whitehead. Since there is almost no opening at the surface, the closed comedo must never be squeezed; in so doing, you would only force its contents deeper into the skin and run the risk of scarring.

OPEN COMEDO. Better known as the blackhead, the open comedo is an acne plug with an opening at the surface. Because of this fact, the contents of the blackhead can usually be emptied by exerting gentle pressure on both of its sides. (Be sure to first steam skin for 15 minutes.) Always use your index fingers, making sure they're wrapped with tissues before you start. (*NOTE*: Never use a "comedo extractor" to remove blackheads, as these instruments can do serious damage to the surrounding skin.) If the material does not come out easily, don't force it! Follow with a dab of 3% hydrogen peroxide on a cotton ball.

Blackheads are not caused by dirt. Their darkish color comes partially from the oxidation of the sebum and partially from the skin's own pigment or melanin. Therefore, blackheads cannot simply be washed away.

PUSTULE. A small red bump that peaks with a yellowish cap of pus is known as a pustule. It is basically a comedo that has ruptured, and when this happens, your body's white blood cells rush in like the infantry to fight the "foreign invaders," which include bacteria, oil, and dead cells.

You may try to drain this type of acne lesion and, if properly done, this process will greatly accelerate the healing of the area. First, make sure your hands are scrupulously clean. Next, sterilize a needle by holding it in the flame of a match for a few seconds. After the needle has cooled, puncture the pustule in the exact center of the yellowish cap. With index fingers wrapped in tissue, gently squeeze the sides of the lesion. Stop when the pus no longer comes out easily. If you force it, you will drive the material deeper into the skin and greatly increase the likelihood of permanent scarring. Now place a warm compress (a clean washcloth soaked in warm water will do) over the area for a few minutes and finish by pressing with a cotton ball dipped in rubbing alcohol.

Warm-water soaks can and should be repeated several times daily until the lesion has healed. The warm water increases the flow of blood to the area and speeds up the healing process.

CYSTIC ACNE. If you have even one acne lesion that resembles a large boil or cyst, you should consider your condition severe and place yourself under the regular care of a qualified cosmetic dermatologist. If finances are worrying you, don't forget that most insurance companies cover acne treatments. Speak with your doctor.

My Step-by-step Method of Treatment

Mine is a multifactored approach to the treatment of acne. Although specific "routes" might vary slightly from patient to patient, in the end "all roads lead to Rome" (that is, clear skin).

STRESS. What better place to start than with a review of one of acne's primary aids and abetters—stress—and to reiterate the extremely detrimental effect it can have on skin. Have you ever experienced a breakout right before an unusually important event, perhaps your wedding or the start of a new job? It is the extra strain put on your emotions by these out-of-the-ordinary occasions that probably caused the blemishes to appear.

The chain of biological events that leads up to a break-out goes like this: Stress activates the hypothalamus gland, which in turn stimulates the pituitary gland. The pituitary sends a message to the adrenal gland indicating that a larger-than-normal number of male hormones (including androgen) should be released immediately. Androgen activates the oil glands to produce sebum, which can result in acne.

I've had cases in which excessive stress has caused patients to pick at blackheads so much that they've ended up creating serious cases of acne for themselves. And I've had one or two who didn't stop there but went on to pick at the scab, causing permanent scarring.

Since a certain amount of stress is simply part of life, and is all right, the key to minimizing its adverse effects lies in the way we handle it. Learning to relax is the obvious solution, but very often this cannot be done by the individual acting alone. If, after thorough examination and testing, I feel that stress is at the root of the problem, I will suggest some form of psychological counseling to resolve the inner conflict.

EXERCISE. In more moderate cases of emotional stress (but ones that are clearly having an adverse effect on the skin), the addition of exercise to the daily routine may prove very beneficial. Not only does exercise stimulate the circulation and aid in the cleansing of the skin (by flushing out impurities through perspiration), it also reduces tension, thus improving one's mental outlook. And a positive outlook cannot be discounted when it comes to creating that "inner glow" so important to a beautiful complexion.

A few words of caution before you start, however. Since exercise does increase the activity of the sweat glands and a buildup of this perspiration can trap oils below the skin, you should always begin your regime with a clean face and shower immediately after you're finished. Whenever possible, wear loose-fitting clothing while you work out, as chafing can aggravate acne on the back and chest. Finally, when selecting a form of exercise, it's wise to keep your choice in the "middle of the road" category—no marathons your first time out, please! Remember, too much of a good thing can sometimes be worse than nothing at all.

REST. Another important acne-combatant is adequate rest. Since the skin repairs and rejuvenates itself while we sleep, the importance of rest to a healthy complexion should be obvious. While needs tend to vary slightly from individual to individual, the standard eight hours per night should suffice for most. What's that you say? You can't possibly devote eight whole hours a day to *just sleeping*? Well, as the old saying goes, if it's really important, you'll find the time for it, and the proper amount of sleep is vital if you want to see an improvement in the condition of your skin.

DIET. "You are what you eat": In my opinion, these are some of the truest words ever spoken. Although the exact correlation between diet and acne remains something of a debate among doctors, I prefer to err on the side of caution. In compliance with this philosophy, I ask that you closely adhere to my basic nutritional program, as well as add the following acne aggravators to your "to be avoided" list:

> All dairy products
>
> Beef (because of the hormones given the animals to fatten them)
>
> Cabbage, shellfish, spinach, artichokes, iodized salt, and kelp (because of the high iodine content of these foods)

VITAMINS AGAINST ACNE. For maximum effectiveness, please incorporate these acne-fighting supplements into your daily vitamin-therapy regime:

○ Vitamin A: 10,000 additional I.U.s. (Not to exceed 20,000 I.U.s unless under a doctor's supervision.)
○ Zinc: an extra 50 mg.
○ Lysine (an amino acid): 500 mg.

Finally, by increasing your daily intake of wheat germ by 2 tablespoons (from 1 to 3), you'll be providing your body with the additional vitamin F it needs to slow down your skin's production of oil.

Guidelines to Non-prescription and Prescription Drugs that Go to Work Immediately

Since acne starts when the cells that line the follicle stick together, instead of sloughing off as they normally do, one way to prevent the disease is to stop the cells from sticking together in the first place.

Fortunately, this can be accomplished. All you need is the proper drying-peeling agent for your skin type and a bit of knowledge regarding its correct usage. Drying-peeling agents work because they contain chemicals that get down *into* the follicle, unlike cleansers and astringents, to peel apart the dead cells that are trying to stick together. These products must be used with great regularity and must be rubbed into the skin.

In order for you to derive maximum benefits from your drying-peeling agent, it is essential that you choose one specifically formulated for your type of skin.

The rating system that follows is a quick and easy way to determine your "range":

What is the texture of your skin?

If it's dry...score 0
If it's normal...score 1
If it's oily ....score 2

What is the tone of your skin?

If it's light ....score 1
If it's medium...score 2
If it's olive or dark ....score 3

What is the severity of your acne?

Fewer than 10 lesions on your face..............score 1
Between 10 and 25 lesions on your face ....score 2
Over 25 lesions on your face or
one large acne cyst...................................score 3

If your total score falls between 1 and 3, you need a mild drying-peeling agent. Between 4 and 6 requires a moderate-strength medication. And a score of 7 or 8 demands a full-strength preparation.

The table below lists the most effective and readily available nonprescription products designed to serve the needs of those in each category.

Mild Medications

Rezamid Acne Lotion
Fostex Medicated Cover-up
Clinique's Anti-Acne Formula

Moderate-strength Medications

Oxy 5*
Acne Aid Lotion
Loroxide Acne Lotion

Full-strength Medications

Saligel
Stridex Maximum Strength Cream Treatment*
Clearasil Super Strength*

THE PROCESS. Start by applying the drying-peeling agent to your face once a day, after washing. Always use a fresh cotton tipped swab or cotton ball, and dispose after each use. Constant touching and retouching of acne lesions with the same instrument makes one highly susceptible to reinfection. To avoid unnecessary irritation of the skin, make sure the area is completely dry before applying the medication (waiting 15 or 20 minutes). Cover areas that are currently broken out, as well as those that have a tendency to be. *But do not cover your entire face!* The T-zone (forehead, nose, and chin) is usually the prime spot for acne, but be sure to avoid placing the medication around the eyes and corners of the mouth, as these areas are much too sensitive for this type of treatment.

*These medications contain benzoyl peroxide—a very effective dry-peeling agent, but some people are allergic to it. Therefore, prior to beginning treatment with a product containing benzoyl peroxide, it is wise to do a patch test. Apply a small amount of the medication—about the size of a quarter—to a portion of the affected area for several consecutive days. If no irritation develops, you can proceed as planned. If, however, you are having an adverse reaction to the product, switch to a formula that contains one (or more) of the other nonprescription chemicals found in drying-peeling agents, including sulfur, resorcinol, and salicylic acid. (Spot coverups should never be confused with drying-peeling agents, for in order to qualify as such, the preparation must contain one or more of the aforementioned chemicals.)

Benzoyl peroxide is a bleaching agent. In order to avoid unwanted lightening of hair, clothes, and pillowcases, allow the product to dry completely before moving on. Finally, avoid products packaged with their own applicator, like Noxema's On-the-Spot. The constant touching and retouching of acne lesions with the same instrument makes one highly susceptible to reinfection. If you must carry medication such as this for the sake of convenience, also take along several disposable cotton-tipped swabs.

IS THE MEDICATION WORKING? You will know if you observe the surface peeling of your skin. Although your skin will appear slightly dry, this drying and peeling action will in no way harm your skin, nor will it cause wrinkles. The only thing you might find discouraging after you start your treatment is the possible appearance of new acne lesions. Believe me when I say that these would have shown up sooner or later. They stem from existing microcomedones, and the peeling action simply brought them to a head a little sooner than would have happened naturally. Remember, the important thing is to prevent new acne plugs from forming.

If your skin appears to be slightly reddened by the use of any acne medication, try applying one of the over-the-counter hydrocortizone cremes to the affected area: Cortaid or Lanacord, for example. This should be done after your drying-peeling agent has dried. The anti-inflammatory properties of these preparations should help to alleviate any minor irritation.

If your skin stops peeling or if your acne gets worse, you may have to alter your plan of action. Sometimes you need to strengthen your acne medication, which can be done in one of two ways: by increasing either the frequency of treatments or the strength of the drying-peeling agent. Never do both at the same time, thinking that if some is good, more is better. It isn't! You will know the change is working when peeling resumes. If the opposite is the case, that is, your medication seems to be too strong, take the reverse tack of decreasing either the frequency of treatments or the strength of the drying-peeling agent.

WINDING DOWN. After your acne has been under control for a period of four to eight weeks, you can begin a maintenance program. Once again, proceed with caution. Change one factor, proceeding one step at a time. Decrease the strength of the peeling agent or, if your acne was severe and you applied your medication twice a day, decrease it to just once. Remain at the lower level for at least two weeks before decreasing another step. Continue this downward progression until your face no longer peels. But if your acne flares up after you decrease your treatment, resume the level at which the condition was under control. Maintain that level until you once again feel confident enough to begin a "slow descent."

RETIN A (VITAMIN A ACID). One drying-peeling agent that requires a prescription is Retin A (tretinoin or retinoic acid, as it's sometimes known). Although the vast majority of acne sufferers will peel with an over-the-counter drying-peeling agent, there are some who will not. For these individuals, vitamin A acid can prove very effective in the clearing of the skin. But, as with any powerful drug, vitamin A acid is not without adverse side effects. Its usage may bring about intense surface peeling as well as extreme irritation in the skin of the patient who applies it too often or incorrectly. For this reason, I insist on close medical supervision of every individual engaged in this form of therapy.

Recently, Retin A has also proven an effective tool in the treatment of aging skin. While it is by no means a replacement for dermabrasion or the chemical peel, it will, through consistent usage, reverse some signs of photoaging (sun damage to the skin which causes premature aging) as well as minimize fine lines and wrinkles but it must be used under medical supervision.

ACCUTANE. Another derivative of vitamin A used to treat very severe cases of cystic acne is the prescription drug accutane. Although touted by some as a wonder drug in treating difficult cases, my opinion is that dangers from the immediate (and unknown long-term) side effects brought on by the drug's usage, do outweigh its possible advantages. Of course, there is always the exception to the rule, but treatment with accutane is something I prescribe only as a last resort. Here are some of the reasons why: The most serious side effect produced by accutane is the documented fact that it can cause birth defects in unborn fetuses. Any woman of childbearing age who is contemplating using the drug should therefore submit to a pregnancy test and be carefully monitored by her doctor throughout the duration of treatment. In addition, accutane frequently causes excessively dry lips, nosebleeds, elevated lipid levels, pains and swelling in the joints and occasional personality changes. Still, as it is sometimes the only thing that will bring really stubborn cases of acne under control, the afflicted individual is often willing to take the risks. Accutane is taken by mouth and the blood must be frequently monitored.

ANTIBIOTICS. The most widely prescribed antibiotic in the treatment of acne is tetracycline, which works by effecting the creation of fatty acids within the follicle. The most common side effect of taking tetracycline is the yeast infection it seems to produce in some women (a risk that can be minimized by adding two extra tablespoons of acidophilus to your daily "beauty cocktail"). Photosensitivity can also be a problem for some people, and tetracycline should be discontinued when going in the sun. If you are taking a multivitamin while on tetracycline, make sure it is a formula that does not contain iron, as that mineral blocks the body's absorption of the drug, and avoid milk.

If tetracycline ceases to be effective in controlling a patient's acne, the doctor will often switch to erythromycin, an antibiotic that works in much the same way. Minocycline is a chemical derivative of tetracycline that has proven effective in some instances when plain tetracycline has failed. The side effects that accompany minocycline can be more severe than those experienced through the usage of tetracycline; one side effect is dizziness.

Sometimes such antibiotics as tetracycline, erythromycin, clindamycin, and lincomycin are used in topical applications with excellent results. The main advantage of a topical over a systemic medicine (one which enters the system) is in the reduced instances of side effects.

BIRTH CONTROL PILLS. When birth control pills were first introduced nearly thirty years ago, they contained very large doses of estrogen and almost always contributed to an improved complexion in acne sufferers. But since estrogens also generated many undesirable side effects, pharmaceutical manufacturers began introducing pills that were formulated with greatly reduced amounts of the hormone. Although these newer pills are easier for most women to take, they do not provide the same degree of relief from acne as did their predecessors. In fact, some formulations may even make the condition worse.

Birth control pills generally thought to help acne are Demulen, Enovid-E, Enovid-5, and Ovulen. Those that usually aggravate the disease include Norinyl, Norlestrin, Ortho-Novum, and Ovral. If you are currently taking one of the formulas believed to worsen acne, speak with your doctor about a possible change in your prescription. (Don't forget to take B-complex vitamins when taking birth control pills.)

INTRALESIONAL STEROID SHOTS. The times when I've felt a kinship to my fellow physicians the obstetricians are the times when I've had a model, actress, or other highly visible individual rushed into my office so that I might administer the "magical injection" that would deliver her to an impending photo shoot or TV commercial, blemish-free. (Fortunately, I've never been called out in the middle of the night for this!) These shots contain a dosage of corticosteroids that is injected directly into the acne lesion. Because the anti-inflammatory properties of cortisone rapidly shrink the blemish, it is usually gone within a couple of days. Occasional dimpling or depression in the skin can occur secondary to these intralesional steroid injections, but fortunately this dimpling is usually reversible and transitory.

Acne Scars Don't Have to Be Forever

I would be greatly remiss to conclude this section without mentioning the wide variety of cosmetic surgery procedures now available to aid in the correction of acne scars. Although I will explain each in the section devoted to cosmetic surgery, I can assure you that there is no need to wear the scars obtained in the heat of your battle with acne. Thanks to the many advances of modern technology, there are several very viable means for virtually eliminating them so that, in the end, "all that's left is the memory." Fortunately for acne sufferers, memories (unlike scars) do tend to fade completely with time!

OILY SENSITIVE SKIN

Like walking a tightrope without the net, learning to manage an oily sensitive skin can prove to be a real balancing act, one that requires both skill and practice to master. Still, with a little extra effort on your part (and some help from the following very soothing suggestions), it can be done!

> Be sure to wash bed linens, face cloths, towels, and any items of personal clothing in a mild, low-sudsing soap such as Ivory. Avoid at all costs regular detergents (which tend to leave a residue) as well as any other harsh products that may come in contact with your skin. If *total* avoidance is simply not possible (when cleaning, for example), protect yourself by wearing rubber gloves.

Never use tissues (such as Kleenex) to remove makeup (or for any other purpose) on your face. They contain fine wood shavings that can easily scratch and irritate delicate skin. Pads of cotton are a much safer alternative.

For facial cleansing, always be sure to use cloths made of 100 percent cotton. You can easily make these yourself by purchasing a package of cloth diapers and cutting them into squares of four. These cloths double as very convenient and soothing masks, if two pieces are alternately dipped in a basin of ice water to which a couple of drops of vinegar have been added. Allow one to rest on your face until the chill has worn off, and then switch to the other piece. Keep doing this for 15 to 20 minutes to calm redness or irritation.

If your complexion is feeling particularly "touchy," avoid any sort of granular exfoliation (that is, one using sugar, salt, or cornmeal). Opt instead for this mask: Mash one papaya and apply to your entire face (and neck, if you wish). The enzyme in this fruit magically and gently "eats" the dead skin cells. You can wash them away in just 20 minutes (using tepid, then cool, water).

Use extra caution when bleaching or waxing facial hair, as this delicate area is very suseptible to problems. To be on the safe side, have it done professionally.

Last but not least, remember to handle your skin as little as possible. Don't rub your face vigorously, and above all, don't scratch it! If itching occurs, place an ice cube in a handkerchief and apply to the area of itching for five or six seconds. The itching will stop!

SKIN DURING PREGNANCY AND MENOPAUSE

Pregnancy and Oily Skin

While oily skin tends to become a bit more so during the first half of pregnancy, the opposite holds true for the second half—a time when most women welcome the boost to their ego a drier complexion can provide.

Be wary, however, of the maternity-vitamin formula you are prescribed. If it's one that contains iodine, discuss the prescription with your doctor. This mineral is a notorious triggerer of acne and should be avoided, even if no current problem exists. I once had to perform a chemodermabrasion on a woman who had lived her entire prepregnancy life virtually blemish-free. Unfortunately, it was not until after she had incurred severe scarring from acne that the culprit (the iodine in her maternity vitamins) was pinpointed.

Menopause

This is a time when the oily-skinned individual often experiences a great improvement in the condition of her complexion (especially if estrogen therapy is employed). However, because the symptoms of menopause can range from slightly annoying to downright hair-raising, some doctors have a tendency to over-prescribe, in an effort to help their patients cope.

Always bear in mind that any medication can have an adverse effect on skin. Before taking it, make sure to weigh the odds. A brisk 30-minute walk each day can do wonders for your state of mind (not to mention your body), so before submitting to chemical mood alteration (i.e. drugs), why not give the physical approach a try by making regular aerobic exercise (jogging, swimming, bicycling or walking) an integral part of your life.

CHANGES TO EXPECT AFTER SIXTY DAYS

Your skin should be much less oily now, with signs of acne markedly decreased.

Your eyes will begin to sparkle around this time, and the whites will be much clearer.

You should also be sleeping like a baby, right through the night!

The Third Thirty Days: Completing the Plan

BODY CARE

You'll find that the skin on your body derives the same positive effects from my anti-aging plan as the skin on your face.

Hands and Feet

Two areas are always a source of concern, regardless of one's skintype: the hands and the feet. For this reason, I'd like to provide you with an overview of preventative care for each.

Over the years, I've seen hundreds of women spend thousands of dollars in an effort to preserve the fresh-faced look of a girl of 25. But a problem occurs when the hands dangling out of their sleeves are decidedly those of a 50-year-old matron. For this reason, if a patient is undergoing a facial cosmetic surgery procedure I will frequently suggest a hand procedure as well.

Unless you are prepared to wear gloves every day for the rest of your life, don't let your hands "give you away." If you follow these simple suggestions, that will never happen:

Keep a bottle of moisturizer next to each sink in your home, and apply it to your hands after every washing.

Wear cotton-lined rubber gloves when submerging your hands in water.

To prevent ugly brown spots from appearing, be sure to include your hands when applying daily sunscreen one half hour before going in the sun. And when temperatures dictate the need for a coat, wear gloves as well.

Hands can also benefit from the masks you use on your face.

Keep your nails neatly manicured; they can be a distinct beauty asset, or a liability, if neglected.

Try massaging an antiperspirant into sweaty palms. This should help to alleviate any potential embarrassment. If you find it irritating, consult your doctor, as there is a new process called ionophoresis that is effective.

Apply moisturizer to hands before going to bed, and, if they're feeling particularly rough and chapped, "lock it in" by wrapping them in a layer of Saran Wrap covered by a pair of white (dyes are potential irritants to skin) cotton gloves. The slight discomfort involved in this procedure is well worth the results it produces.

Our feet really take a beating each day, which is why nature provided us with an extra thick protective sole. However, if left unattended, the skin in this area becomes extremely thick, tough, and generally unattractive. Regularity of care is the key to prevent this from happening. If you follow these simple guidelines every day, your feet will keep you "walking on air" for the rest of your life:

At the end of the day, fill a small plastic basin with warm soapy water (you may prefer to use bath oil) and give your feet a good soak for at least 15 minutes (longer, if time permits).

Pat dry and go over any rough, calloused areas (such as heels) with a pumice stone. For stubborn callouses, try standing in an inch or two of bleach, which will have a softening effect. Pat dry after one minute and apply a good moisturizer.

Lavish with moisturizer and, one night a week (more if you wish), wrap your feet in Saran Wrap, as suggested for the hands, substituting white cotton socks for gloves.

It's also an excellent idea to prop your legs up with a couple of pillows and relax for 20 minutes each day. This reverses the pull of gravity your feet and legs are constantly exposed to and gives them a much-needed "breather."

Finally, be sure to change shoes, from high heels to low, very often. This relieves the calf muscles and keeps the Achilles tendon from becoming shortened.

Acne on the Back

Acne on the back is a frequent complaint. It seems to affect a wide cross-section of individuals of all skintypes. Here's the best way for everyone to bring it under control:

Always use a back brush and mild soap to properly cleanse the area during your daily shower or bath.

After the area is thoroughly dry, apply a slightly stronger drying-peeling agent (say, 10 percent benzoyl peroxide) than you'd use on your face. This suggestion is made because of the difficulty involved in reapplication of the product. (Thorough coverage of the area requires the aid of another person. If you live alone, just do the best that you can.)

Since it is not necessary to wash the area before the agent is applied, apply it once in the morning and once before retiring.

To boost your efforts, try any one of the masks for oily skin (listed in that section) on the back. Apply, let dry for 20 minutes and shower off.

If the acne on your back is very severe, it may be necessary for you to add another bath or shower to your daily routine, at least until the condition has been brought under control. (Don't forget to remoisturize dry areas of the body immediately afterwards.) And always remember to shower immediately after any activity which has caused you to perspire. (It's best to wear absorbant clothing during aerobic work-outs.)

Finally, if all of your attempts to bring the condition under control fail, consult a dermatologist before scarring occurs. Some problems of this nature are very stubborn and will respond only to prescription-strength medication.

Warning: These Ingredients May Be Hazardous to the Health of Your Skin

The following is a list of potential irritants to oily skin commonly found in treatment products, moisturizers and foundations. Although they may not bother you now, skins *do* change. For this reason, always check the label of every new product before you buy it, especially if your skin is feeling particularly sensitive.

- ❍ Detergents such as sodium lauryl sulfate & laureth-4
- ❍ Isopropyl myristate
- ❍ Isopropyl palmitate
- ❍ Isopropyl isostearate
- ❍ Butyl stearate
- ❍ Isostearyl neopentanoate
- ❍ Cetyl oleate
- ❍ Octyl palmitate
- ❍ Isocetyl stearate
- ❍ Lanolin
- ❍ Preservatives

SUN SPECIFICS

Aging's first lieutenant in the field, the sun is beauty's greatest natural enemy, even for those with thicker, oily skin. Although total avoidance is your only secure defense, it would be difficult to imagine a life lived entirely on the "inside." In lieu of that approach, here are some of the most effective ways I've found to minimize the negative effects of the sun:

Get into the sunscreen habit. Apply one with an SPF of at least 15 every morning, alone or under makeup one half hour before exposure to the sun. (With SPF 15 protection, the skin can tolerate the sun 15 times longer than without a protective product. With SPF 4, 4 times longer, etc.) I believe a sunscreen of SPF 15 or 20 is about the most effective you can get today. More than that is just wishful thinking.

To protect the areas that are among the first to show signs of aging, always include hands and neck in your sunblock coverage.

Because the skin on your lips contains very little melanin, this area requires SPF protection of its own. Make sure it gets it by regularly using one of the "lip blocks" on the market, either alone or under your lipstick. (By the way, the brighter the shade, the better the protection.) Remember to reapply frequently whenever you're out in the sun, and always after eating or drinking.

Don't forget your sunglasses. Wear them twelve months of the year! Best are the wraparound kind and ones that indicate their UV (Ultra Violet) protection. To further shield this delicate area, use one of the sunblocks created specifically for use around eyes.

Hats (especially the wide-brimmed variety) are always in style when it comes to spending a day in the sun.

Avoid taking PABA by mouth. Taken orally, it frequently incites a negative reaction in the skin.

Don't believe the ads: Sun beds and tanning booths are every bit as detrimental to skin as the real thing.

All of the following can make you extrasensitive to sun. If you must be in it, avoid them:

Many medications, including antibiotics, birth control pills, diuretics, and tranquilizers. Check with your doctor to see if anything else you might be taking applies.

Germicidal soaps and antiseptics that contain hexachlorophene and bithionol.

Any product that's alcohol based, such as astringent, perfume, after-shave, and cologne.

Excessive amounts of vitamins A and C. (More than 20,000 I.U.s of vitamin A a day or more than 2,000 mgs of vitamin C a day.)

Remember: *Be afraid of your own shadow*! It's there to remind you that the sun's damaging rays are lurking close by.

CHANGES TO EXPECT AFTER NINETY DAYS

Your skin should have completely normalized by now, with all signs of active acne gone.

All surface facial wrinkles will have virtually disappeared, making you look substantially younger than you did a short three months ago.

Skin on the backs of your hands will have tightened significantly at this point, making them much more youthful in appearance.

Your energy level will be at its peak. You'll feel on top of the world and never more alert!

My Ninety-Day ☐ Plan for Combination Skin

If you're like most people with combination skin, you've probably spent half your life praying for the day when a truce would be called and the two sides of your face would unite into one. Although at its best combination skin is considered about as normal as any complexion can be, at its worst it may require a full-time "referee"!

Generally, combination skin ages slightly more gracefully than dry skin and not quite as well as oily complexions. But now, through my extraordinary plan, there's no longer a need for any distinction among skintypes. For everyone who follows the program, the end result is the same: simply beautiful skin!

Highly motivated and very successful in her career as a stockbroker, Alison W.'s naturally aggressive style had always proven a tremendous professional asset. Unfortunately, the same approach was a liability when it was applied to the handling of her skin. Although in her late 40s, Alison still practiced the extremely harsh and drying regimen of skincare she'd started during her acne-plagued adolescence.

Time had finally caught up with her, as the years of cumulative abuse manifested themselves in topskin dryness, a condition characterized by excessive flakiness and a generally dull appearance. The skin's surface layers become so parched that they camouflage the healthy skin lying just beneath.

I urged that Alison immediately embark on my anti-aging program for dry skin, asking that she continue to adhere to its guidelines until all traces of flakiness had disappeared, in, I estimated, approximately sixty days.

Sure enough, within two months an entirely new Alison returned to my office. Gone were all signs of the topskin dryness and in its place was a rapidly normalizing and increasingly beautiful complexion.

At that point, I advised her to switch to my plan for the combination skin. And, with a complexion that's completely normalized as well as free of blemishes and wrinkles, there she happily remains, four years and innumerable compliments later!

A former Miss America, Mary's smooth, wrinkle-free complexion and lithe figure belie the twenty years that have gone by since she won the crown. But that was not always the case.

Just two years ago, a decidedly more mature-looking Mary had come to see me in search of a cure for the cumulative damage years of unprotected sunworshipping had inflicted on her skin. Of particular concern were the ever-deepening lines and spots of hyperpigmentation (skin discolorations) such overexposure had caused to appear on her face, her neck, and the backs of her hands. And although *these* areas were excessively dry, her T-zone had remained oily, occasionally even breaking out in attacks of acne.

To make matters worse, Mary had recently undertaken an overzealous (and medically unsupervised) regimen of Retin A therapy in an attempt to eradicate some of the damage herself. Unfortunately, it was a move that served only to add irritation to her already troubled complexion.

After assuring her that her ''beauty prime'' had been written off far too prematurely, I outlined a plan through which it could be restored. I included an overview of my advanced vitamin and nutrition therapies, as well as an outline of my simple, step-by-step regimen for the proper daily care of her combination skin.

Elated by the possibilities the program held for her, Mary left the office that day full of enthusiasm and hope. She later confided she'd felt as though she'd just been handed a renewed lease on youth (which, in fact, she had)! Within only three months, Mary was back, proudly displaying the fruits of her efforts.

Virtually gone were the crow's feet and other unbecoming facial lines she'd found so disconcerting, as well as all signs of acne and the redness and irritation she'd recently experienced. In their place was a moist, youthful radiance and evenness of tone she thought her complexion had lost forever.

As an added bonus to the plan, Mary was delighted to report an effortless fifteen-pound weight loss—one she'd been trying, without success, to achieve for more than five years.

But perhaps the biggest reward and boost to her ego came with her return to the Miss America Pageant, her first appearance at the Atlantic City event in more than a decade. Mary couldn't hide her sheer delight as she told me of the frequency with which she was mistaken for one of the current contestants!

Mary has remained a devout follower of my natural approach and has "beauty queen" good looks (along with an impressive array of sun hats and glasses) to show for it today.

The cases described are only two of the hundreds I've treated involving people: individuals who could never envision their combination skins as anything more than what they presently were (and had always been) to them—strictly double trouble.

Shortly after beginning my anti-aging plan, these same patients began to perceive their complexions in an entirely new and expanded light. By the ninety-day mark, none of them so much as mentioned the word "skintype," but they couldn't stop talking about beautiful skin—their own!

With everything you need to follow in their footsteps contained in the pages of this section, why delay another minute in getting started? Remember, there's a flawless complexion in you just waiting to be revealed. Don't make the wait too long!

My Ninety-Day Plan for Combination Skin

The First Thirty Days: De-aging the Skin

DAILY CARE

Your personal care, every day, is the most important element in maintaining beautiful, young-looking skin; without a meticulously cared-for complexion, one can never hope to fulfill one's true beauty potential. With this in mind, I've developed the following "natural alternatives" to more traditional treatment products. Created especially for use on combination skin, the formulas are all very easy to prepare, inexpensive, and extremely effective. Once you've tried them and seen for yourself the difference they can make, I'm certain you'll never use another thing on your face.

Here is your program of daily care:

Morning

STEP 1: CLEANSING. Apply 2 to 3 tablespoons of plain natural yogurt (very soothing) to damp skin and massage well over face and neck (concentrating on the T-zone—the forehead, nose and chin). Follow with 20 splashes of warm water to insure that no residue remains on the skin.

STEP 2: TONING. After cleansing, stir 1 teaspoon of apple cider vinegar into an 8-ounce glass of water (more if skin is very sensitive). Apply only to T-zone with pads of cotton and in an upward sweeping motion. This recipe can be doubled or tripled and stored in a tightly closed bottle or jar in refrigerator.

STEP 3: NOURISHING. While skin is still damp, lock in moisture by applying one of the three nourishing alternatives that follow. Confine their application to dry areas of the face.

Either: A thin layer of margarine (the kind sold in health food stores) that contains no artificial colorings, flavorings, or preservatives. (Amazingly, when topically applied, the margarine sinks right into skin, leaving no greasy residue.)

Or: A light application of *mayonnaise*. To insure its quality, try making it yourself, using the following recipe:

> To 1 slightly beaten egg yolk, add a cup of olive oil, 1 teaspoon at a time. When the mixture starts to thicken, whisk in 1 teaspoon of fresh lemon juice, and voilà—the "makings" of smooth skin! Mayonnaise can be stored like the toner, but only for four or five days. Restir before each usage.

Or: If mayonnaise or margarine don't appeal to you, a light application of olive or any cold-pressed oil is also good.

Evening

STEP 1: MAKEUP REMOVAL. Any thin, natural, cold-pressed oil may be used for this purpose, with avocado, olive, and safflower oils all registering as popular choices. Simply massage oil lightly over the face and throat, removing it with pads of damp cotton. Repeat until the last traces of both oil and makeup have disappeared.

STEP 2: CLEANSING. Same as in the morning.

STEP 3: EXFOLIATING. Necessary for removing the dead cell accumulation that naturally occurs on all types of skin, this procedure is most beneficial when performed on a daily basis. Several readily available products may be used for exfoliating, including sea salt, yellow cornmeal, and sugar. The latter also benefits skin by having a slightly antibacterial effect.

To make a paste, start by adding a teaspoon of water to a small amount of any one of the three ingredients; gradually increasing the moisture content until a desired consistency is reached. Then, *gently* scrub the mixture over the entire face and throat area with tips of fingers to loosen debris from the surface of pores. Finish by rinsing well with warm water, followed by a cool splash.

STEP 4: TONING. Same as in the morning.

STEP 5: NOURISHING. Same as in the morning.

Extra Help:

MASKS. To enhance the effects of any mask, gently steam your face before applying. Simply toss a few bags of chamomile tea into a pot of boiling water, remove from the stove, and, draping a towel over your head in a tentlike fashion, capture the steam.

Masks should be made fresh for each use.

The masks you can make yourself are every bit as effective, and varied, as those you can buy. Remember always to apply to a clean skin and try to use a mask once or twice a week. Here are some of the very best masks I've found in treating the combination complexion. Incidentally all masks listed in both oily and dry skin sections may be applied to the oily and dry parts of your face.

> "Two in One" Egg Mask. Perfect for combination skin, the incredibly versatile egg is an individually wrapped, custom-designed facial mask! To take advantage of its remarkable abilities, simply separate the egg and beat the two parts individually. Cover the oily areas of your face with the white and the drier parts with the yolk. Allow to remain for 20 minutes. Remove with warm water.

> For a super clarifying treatment. Combine 1 tablespoon of almonds (finely ground in blender) with the same amount of honey and 1 egg white. Allow to dry on face for 15 to 20 minutes. Remove by massaging with warm water in a rotating motion over skin. Rinse well.

> For a quick pick-me-up. Mix together 1 ounce each of orange and lemon juice and then fold in the white of an

TOPICAL TREATMENTS AND WHY THEY WORK SO WELL

Apple cider vinegar. Restores skin to proper pH (acid/alkaline) balance.

Lemon. Rich in vitamin C, potassium, and iron, it gives tone to the skin and acts as a mild bleach.

Nail-polish remover. When applied with cotton-tipped swab to *individual blemishes only*, the acetone it contains rapidly dries up the lesions, thus accelerating the healing process.

Oatmeal or Wheatena. Gently exfoliates and deep-cleanses the skin. It also soothes irritations.

Vodka. As a very pure form of alcohol, it is a very effective astringent for tightening pores.

White sugar. An extremely efficient skin exfoliant, with the added advantage of having a slightly antibacterial effect on the complexion.

Yogurt. Cleanses and soothes the skin; reduces visible signs of irritation.

Milk of magnesia. Has a very healing effect on acne. Since it is slightly drying to the skin, its usage should be confined to individual lesions only.

egg, beating the mixture until it is frothy. Allow your skin to "drink it in" for 20 minutes! Remove with warm water.

For intensive moisturizing of dry patches. Prepare a well-beaten egg yolk with 1 teaspoon of olive oil and apply to the skin. Leave in place for 10 minutes. After that time, spread a stiffly beaten egg white evenly over the first mixture and allow to dry for another 15 minutes before removal.

For a relaxing (dry skin) massage. For a dry, dehydrated skin, heat ½ cup of peanut oil until warm and massage into face and neck. Remove excess by blotting with a clean tissue.

For loosening black heads. Cook 1 ounce of barley with enough water to cover, until soft. Apply to skin while still warm and allow to remain for 15 minutes. Remove with a damp soft cloth or by splashing with warm water.

TO HYDRATE THE SKIN. Dehydrated skin generally appears blotchy and responds well to the addition of moisture (water, not oil).

Any type of skin can become dehydrated, given the right set of circumstances. For intense skin rehydration, such as is needed after overexposure to the elements, I've found the following treatment unbeatable:

Apply predigested liquid protein with soluble collagen (the kind once used, rather dangerously, for dieting and still available at most health food stores) to face and neck. (A wooden tongue depressor—available at most drug stores—is useful for evenly spreading the liquid.) Allow to dry and remain on skin for 1 or 2 hours, lightly spritzing the area with water at 15- to 20-minute intervals. Rinse well after allotted time has passed. The hydrating effect this has on skin seems to last for several days following application.

TO DRY ACNE LESIONS. Apply nail-polish remover directly onto the blemish with a cotton-tipped swab. The acetone in the formula will aid in drying up the lesion. (*One note*: As some nail-polish removers are now acetone-free, be sure to check for this ingredient before purchasing for this purpose.)

Milk of magnesia applied in the same manner will produce a similar effect; its less-harsh formula makes it a wiser choice for those with more sensitive skin.

TO REDUCE PUFFINESS AROUND EYES. *Either*: Obtain 2 slices from inside of potato and place over closed eyes. Rest in this position for 15 minutes prior to applying makeup.

Or: Use tea bags that have been dipped in hot water and then chilled. Apply in the same manner. Incidentally, the cheaper brands of tea are usually highest in tannic acid, the ingredient that produces the desired effect.

Or: Sleep on two or three pillows at night.

TO REDUCE UNDER-EYE BAGS. Cut a raw fig in half and place a section over each eye. Keeping them closed, relax for 20 minutes.

TO FADE RED SPOTS ON SKIN. Combine 1 tablespoon each of freshly squeezed lemon juice and salt. Using a cotton-tipped swab, place mixture directly on reddened areas. After 10 minutes, rinse well.

NUTRITION AND VITAMIN THERAPY

Building Strength from Within

Have you ever heard anyone ask, "Is it surgery or sardines?" as they pondered the reason for someone's particularly young, attractive appearance? While the answer to that query could be a combination of the two, you may not be aware of the significant role the lowly sardine can play in maintaining beautiful skin.

On the anti-aging nutritional team, the sardine could easily be voted most valuable player, for this humble fish has the profound distinction of being the only food to double its already high content of RNA (ribonucleic acid) and DNA (deoxyribonucleic acid) while in the can.

RNA and DNA are the "stuff cells are made of." And cells— by the millions—are the things that make up our bodies, each with a lifespan of approximately two years. Before the cell dies, it reproduces itself on orders given by a commander-in-chief (DNA) and carried out by a messenger (RNA). In theory, therefore, we should look the same today as we did ten or fifteen years ago. But unfortunately, as with most theories, this one has holes in it.

Because of a variety of external factors beyond our control, the cell goes through some deterioration with each successive reproduction, causing an alteration in its shape. The further away it moves from its original blueprint, the more visibly we show signs of aging.

Interestingly and very encouragingly, however, the matter is not entirely out of our hands. Work pioneered by the late Benjamin Frank, M.D. demonstrated that if we keep our bodies well supplied with external sources of the nucleic acids (like sardines), we can rejuvenate the cells to the point where the aging process is drastically retarded or even reversed. In addition, we will be contributing to an overall improvement in appearance as well as to a general sense of well-being. And therein lies the basis for my anti-aging nutritional plan, which will, if carefully followed, change much more than simply the way you eat.

So if you're ready to start feeling stronger, thinking more clearly, aging more slowly, and looking much, much better, I invite you to proceed to the specifics of the plan.

My Anti-aging Nutritional Plan*

Four days per week, have a 3 or 4 ounce can of sardines.

Three other days per week, have one of the following: a serving of salmon, tuna, sole, bluefish, scrod or monk-fish.

Once or twice a week, have a serving of liver (chicken liver is best).

Have 2 or 3 eggs each week, if your cholesterol level is not elevated. (If this is a question, check with your doctor.)

Everyday, include 1 serving of fresh pineapple or papaya, in addition to 1 serving of any other fresh fruit.

Twice a week, have a serving of lentils, peas, lima beans, or soybeans, as well as a serving of avocado.

Each day, have a salad prepared with some or all of the following ingredients: spinach, mushrooms, onions, asparagus, radishes, celery, scallions, beets, carrots, and broccoli.

Have 1 tablespoon each of bran, wheat germ, brewer's yeast, and lecithin granules daily.

Two or three times per week, have a serving of oatmeal or Wheatena.

Include in your daily beverage intake all of the following: 1 glass fruit or vegetable juice; 2 glasses of skimmed milk; and 6 to 8 glasses (8 oz.) of pure (preferably bottled) water.

Have oat bran muffins for breakfast frequently. It lowers cholesterol and is great for fiber.

*If you are currently under a physician's care, check with your doctor before embarking on this or any other specialized nutritional program.

Finally, to detoxify your system and keep it running smoothly, enjoy this daily ''beauty cocktail'': Mix 3 tablespoons liquid acidophilus (friendly bacteria) and 1 tablespoon lactose into an 8-ounce glass of water, and drink to good health . . . yours! (You can buy both acidophilus and lactose in your local health food store.) The good bacteria in this cocktail will help destroy and eliminate toxins from the body.

If you stick strictly to this diet—with no additions—you'll lose weight. If weight is not a problem for you, the aforementioned foods may be incorporated into your regular diet, provided it does not include any of the following foods which, must be *avoided*. If this proves to be too difficult, certainly try to *minimize* them in your diet.

Anything containing white flour or sugar; for sweetening, small amounts of honey or blackstrap molasses make healthy alternatives.

Alcoholic beverages; try a sparkling water like Perrier or Pellegrino and lemon or lime instead.

Red meat; dark poultry meat is all right.

Salt; garlic can be used in many instances as a substitute.

Fats; cold-pressed oils, such as safflower, are permitted in moderation.

Products containing caffeine; herbal teas are fine.

Bringing on the Reinforcements

Each day, include the following vitamin and mineral supplements in your diet:

One high-potency multivitamin containing chelated minerals after breakfast. (''Chelated'' is your key to no stomach upset from certain supplements. Look for it on labels.)

One RNA/DNA tablet (125 mg.) after lunch. (Not to exceed daily intake of 150 mg.—including multivitamins.)

Two high-potency B-complex vitamin tablets, one after breakfast and one after lunch. (Not to exceed total daily intake—including multivitamin—of 100 mg. of each of the following: Vit. B-1, Vit. B-2, Vit. B-6, Vit. D, and 100 mcg. of Vit. B-12, 400 mcg. of folic acid and 300 mcg. of Biotin

Two vitamin C tablets with bioflavinoids (500 mg. each), one after eating. (Not to exceed total daily intake—including multivitamin—of 1,000 mg.) Higher doses may cause stomach upset.

Vitamin E (800 I.U.s, dry form) once a day after breakfast. (Not to exceed total daily intake including multivitamin of 800 I.U.s)

Selenium (100 mcg.) once a day, taken in conjunction with vitamin E. (Not to exceed daily intake of 100 mcg.—including multivitamin.)

Vitamin A (10,000 I.U.s) daily after lunch. (Not to exceed total daily intake—including multivitamin—of 20,000 I.U.s)

Chelated zinc (50 mcg.) daily after breakfast. (Not to exceed intake of 100 mg.—including multivitamin)

Cysteine, an amino acid (500 mg.), midafternoon with a glass of either orange or grapefruit juice. (Not to exceed intake of 500 mg. daily—including multivitamin)

If this seems like a lot to swallow, imagine what a bitter pill it would be to discover, too late, that many of your blemishes, lines, and wrinkles were preventable.

Putting the Plan into Action for You

What follows is an outline of a typical day on my anti-aging nutritional plan.

BREAKFAST

High-energy shake made with:

  8 ounces skim milk
  ½ cup fresh raspberries

1 tablespoon each, brewer's yeast and lecithin granules
Honey, to taste
2–3 ice cubes (for thickness)

Mix on high speed in blender until frothy.

Bowl of cooked oatmeal sprinkled with 1 tablespoon each of bran and wheat germ.

Herbal tea

After breakfast, the following supplements:

1 high-potency multivitamin/multimineral
1 vitamin B-complex tablet
500 mg. vitamin C with bioflavinoids
800 I.U.s vitamin E (dry form)
100 mcg. selenium
50 mg. chelated zinc

SUGGESTED FOODS AND HOW THEY BENEFIT YOUR SYSTEM

Sardines. Highest single source of nucleic acids (RNA/DNA). The only food to double such content while in the can.

Oatmeal or Wheatena. Also a good source of RNA/DNA, as well as natural fiber. When paired with bran, has been shown to be effective in reducing levels of cholesterol.

Papaya. Contains valuable digestive properties as well as valuable nutrients.

Lentils. Excellent alternate source of protein; also rich in nucleic acid.

Lecithin. Used in the making of chocolate to keep it from hardening before its time; has a similar effect on one's arteries. Also, an important moisture-binding agent.

Yogurt. Furnishes useful bacteria that keep the intestines clean by countering toxic substances.

The reason for one firm "no no"—alcohol. Especially when taken with meals, it tends to raise levels of uric acid, the very thing the diet strives to prevent by emphasizing fluids.

LUNCH

Cup of borscht (beet soup, served hot or cold)

Large spinach salad (including mushrooms, onions, and a hard-boiled egg), topped with a tablespoon each of safflower oil and red-wine vinegar

Serving of fresh pineapple

Perrier and lime

After lunch, these supplements:

> 125 mg. RNA/DNA tablet
> 10,000 I.U.s vitamin A
> 1 vitamin B-complex tablet

MIDAFTERNOON

> 500 mg. cysteine with 4 ounces of grapefruit juice

DINNER

½ avocado with lemon

Bouillabaisse (Mixed-seafood stew)

Small green salad

Dish of strawberries (fresh)

Herbal tea

After dinner, this supplement:

> 500 mg. vitamin C with bioflavinoids

BEFORE BED

> Glass of skimmed milk

If weight is not a problem for you, the aforementioned meals may be augmented as you wish, excluding, of course, the foods on the "to be avoided" roster.

Last, but not least, be creative! And remember to view each and every dining experience as the wonderfully rejuvenating treat for your skin that it is.

Sardine "Surprises"

Sardines are an amazingly versatile (not to mention incredibly healthy) food that should be eaten often. Here are a few innovative ways to maximize their appeal:

Peppers Stuffed with Sardines

2 large green peppers
3½ oz. can sardines (water packed), chopped
1 cup cooked rice
1½ medium-sized onion, minced
½ cup tomato sauce
1 egg
Salt and pepper

With a paring knife, cut a circle around the stem of each pepper. Pull out the stems, and, with a fork or teaspoon, scrape away as many of the seeds from the hollow as you can. Rinse them out with cold water.

Mix the sardines with the rice, the onion, and the tomato sauce. Beat the egg and add this along with approximately ½ teaspoon of salt and a dash of pepper.

Put this mixture into the hollow peppers, and bake for about 20 minutes at 350°F.

Sardines with Gouda Cheese

This makes a superb easy-to-cook main dish for two.

2 3½ oz. cans sardines
1 pound spinach
1½ cup skimmed milk
3 tablespoons corn oil margarine
3 tablespoons flour
2 teaspoons Worcestershire sauce
¾ cup crumbled Gouda cheese

Drain the sardines into a large frying pan, and set the sardines aside.

Wash the spinach and tear it into bite-sized pieces. Heat the sardine oil and pile spinach onto it. Cover and cook over low heat for 5 minutes, until the margarine melts.

While the spinach is cooking put 1 cup of the skimmed milk into a saucepan with the margarine. Heat over very low heat until the margarine melts.

Mix the flour into the rest of the skimmed milk, and pour the mixture slowly into the heating milk while stirring. Add the Worcestershire sauce, and all but 3 tablespoons of the cheese. Continue stirring until cheese melts, making sure the mixture does not boil.

Put the cooked spinach into a greased baking dish. Then place the sardines on top of the spinach and the cheese sauce on top of everything. Sprinkle the rest of the cheese on this, and bake at 400°F until the cheese melts (about 10 minutes).

A Canapé

Very lightly toast 2 slices of white bread. Cut each slice into 4 pieces. Mash 3½ ounces of sardines with a fork and spread over the bread pieces. Top with a few shavings of Swiss cheese and bake at 350°, until the cheese melts.

COMBATING THE SABOTEURS OF YOUNG SKIN

The time bandits that fall into this category have been guilty of bringing on an "early frost" in more cases than I'd care to mention, so let's examine the ways in which each of them contribute to the skin's demise and what can be done to minimize the damage.

For starters, you have an extremely powerful ally in your running battle with time, running right out of your kitchen and bathroom faucets! That's right, good old H_2O can be your single best defense when it comes to beating the clock, so be sure to take full advantage. Since, however, one can never be sure of the quality of tap water, it's best to either install a charcoal filter or drink the bottled variety.

The following are some of water's many and varied uses. I strongly suggest you immediately incorporate each of them into your daily life:

> Increase your consumption of the liquid by having at least 1 quart each day. This will aid in the removal of toxins from your system, which in turn will prevent them from having a negative impact on your skin (especially important for clearing a blemished complexion). Keep a pitcher of chilled water in the refrigerator at all

times. For a refreshing and slightly tangy change of pace, try adding a few slices of fresh lemon to the container before storing.

If you haven't done so already, purchase a humidifier and keep it going in your bedroom while you sleep. It's a small investment that will pay big dividends in moisture restored to your skin. (Be sure to change the water daily.) If you rely on a humidifier instead of additional lubricant to keep your complexion moist at night, you'll substantially lessen the risk of "overnourishing" your skin.

When washing your face, always rinse with twenty splashes of tepid water. Rehydrate often throughout the day by "spritzing" the area with one of the mineral waters (Evian, for example) sold in an aerosol can. This is especially important when traveling by air, as the pressurized cabins are extremely drying to skin. For the same reason, make your cocktails Perrier or another bottled water instead of alcohol.

Sun

Because of the overwhelmingly negative impact the sun has on skin, I've devoted an entire section to the topic ("Sun specifics" in "The Third Thirty Days: Completing the Plan,") for your enlightenment. Precautions should be taken at all times—no matter what the weather. But if you are planning a vacation to the tropics where exposure is imminent, extra precautions should be taken.

Exposure

When it comes to the aging effects of the elements (wind, heat, cold), total avoidance is your best defense. Unfortunately, from the day you leave the hospital in your mother's arms, this is a virtually impossible task, so the next best thing is to always take the proper precautions. Be sure to apply a sunscreen with an SPF of at least 15 to your face, neck, (alone or under make-up) and backs of the hands each morning; wear sunglasses all year round whenever exposed to the sun, regardless of the temperature; wear protective clothing (i.e. heat reflecting for summer and insulated for winter, including hat and gloves.)

Now when I speak of "the elements," you probably think this refers only to the ones we're exposed to out of doors. On the contrary, the seasonal accommodations we make indoors (central heating and air conditioning) are every bit as detrimental to the health of your skin as their fresh-air counterparts. (Remember, it's water, not oil, that keeps skin moist.) Therefore, environmental protection on both fronts is definitely in order. Don't forget the humidifier. This is especially important in winter. And keep plants around—they're good for your skin!

Make certain your skincare routine changes whenever your wardrobe does. Winter's cold and gusty winds are far more drying to skin than summer's heat and humidity, so be certain to cleanse, tone, and moisturize accordingly.

Facial Stress

Squinting, sneering, scowling, pursing the lips, knitting the brow—all are common, everyday habits that happen to be major contributing factors to a condition known as facial stress: the self-inflicted damage done to facial muscles through chronic grimacing and general fatigue.

Although these reflexes are in some cases deeply ingrained in the mannerisms of an individual, for most people an awareness of their existence is usually all it takes to arrest the problem. A patient once came to see me requesting collagen injections in the furrows of her brow. After noting the wrinkle-free appearance of the rest of her face, I advised that she might unconsciously be causing or aggravating the lines. To verify this fact, I suggested that she place a mirror on her desk at work and one near her telephone at home.

By setting up a "wrinkle watch" in this manner, she became aware that she was fervently knitting her brow during every telephone conversation. Once the collagen injections had corrected the problem, I suggested she might avoid a recurrence by placing small strips of hair-setting tape over the susceptible areas while at home. The slight tightening effect this produced at every twist and turn served as a more than sufficient deterrent whenever her face decided to "go into motion."

The same technique can be applied to any area of the face that is noticeably more lined than the rest. By closely observing the bad habits you probably didn't even realize you had, you can usually put a stop to them and, hence, the damage that results.

Now that you know how to stop these facial distortions "in their tracks" (or hopefully before they've left any permanent ones on your face), here are some other ways they get their start:

Smoking is a double offender. Inhaling entails the pursing of the lips, while exhaling causes the eyes to squint (a reaction of self-defense to prevent the smoke from entering). In addition, smoking depletes the body's supply of Vitamin C, vital for its production of collagen.

Another frequent cause of squinting is poor vision. To avoid this problem, see your ophthalmologist regularly, and keep your prescription for corrective lenses up to date.

Making a concerted effort to get all the sleep you need (for most this means the standard eight hours per night) can be a great beauty boon, as a lack of sleep really does "show on your face." Skin cells repair and rejuvenate themselves during periods of slumber, so opt for nine hours whenever possible.

Try training yourself to sleep on your back (or at least start the night out in that position). It just might help put an end to the formation of lines and wrinkles that are a result of your face pressing against the pillow night after night. (Satin-cased pillows are best, by the way.)

The Use and Abuse of Alcohol

In addition to dehydrating the system and depleting the body's supply of the B vitamins, long-term consumption of alcohol can lead to dilation of the blood vessels. Eventually this can result in a condition known as rosacea, which gives the nose a red, blotchy, bulbous appearance. And let's face it, no matter how popular a nostalgia craze becomes, you might long for Cleopatra's eyes and adore Mona Lisa's smile, but one look no one will ever want is that of W. C. Fields's nose (the most famous case of rosacea)! If you're not already "on the wagon," for your skin's sake please climb aboard.

Emotional Stress

It flushes with embarrassment and rage, and it blanches with fear. There's no doubt about it, your skin truly is your body's emotional barometer.

If you have any doubt about just how aging chronic stress can be, compare two photographs of almost any official elected to high public office: one taken upon entering, the other on leaving the job. Such an image is worth more than a thousand words of warning. I treat many of these individuals, and, as a group, they challenge my skills for holding time at bay more than any other.

Since, however, stress is a fact of life that can never be completely eliminated, we must find a way (anything from self-hypnosis to psychotherapy) of handling it. The important thing is to discover a relaxation technique that works for you and to practice it regularly.

Lack of Exercise

Besides being a great source of stress relief (especially the aerobic variety), exercise flushes impurities out of the system through perspiration, improves circulation by carrying increased oxygen to cells, and firms and tones the muscles. It should therefore be apparent to even the greatest skeptic that exercise plays the vital role in postponing the visible signs of aging. Exercise is the body's true fountain of youth.

If you're not currently engaged in a regular sport—whether it be walking, jogging, swimming, or bicycling—find an activity you enjoy, start slowly, and build up the pace. Three times a week for at least one half hour is essential for cardio-pulmonary function as well as terrific skin. The vast improvement in the way you look and feel will serve as more than sufficient incentive for continuing.

In addition, you can reverse the pull of gravity, to a certain extent, by standing on your head or lying on a slantboard with your feet elevated for ten minutes each day. (Any 6- to 8-foot-long plank of wood—at least 10 inches wide—can be used.) Along with increasing the flow of blood to the dermis (creating a glow in the complexion), this action is an excellent energizer! (*A word of warning*: This position can cause extra pressure on the eyes. For those who are predisposed to conditions such as glaucoma, it could create or aggravate a problem. It is therefore best to check with your doctor before beginning.)

Rapid and Frequent Changes in Weight

If you abuse your body by subjecting it to the "yo-yo" dieting syndrome, you are doing your skin more of a disservice than if you remained consistently overweight. The skin's elasticity is by no means "snap-proof," and if the body's supply of fat is constantly being depleted and restored, its resiliency simply wears out. Left with improper support, the irreversibly stretched skin can be likened to a tent at the end of camping season, once you've collapsed the pole; the canvas is left to drape loosely over whatever remains.

Early in my career, I treated one such individual. Anna P. first came to see me to discuss ways in which her sagging facial skin (the result of a 100-pound weight loss) could be tightened. Although, as I suspected, it was the same 100 pounds she had gained and lost countless times before, she assured me that this time the loss was permanent. Besides having maintained her current weight for close to four years, she said she now held an executive position with the weight-loss organization that had inspired her success and was under constant pressure there to stay thin. She felt the current state of her skin made her look a good twenty years older than she really was, and I agreed.

Several weeks following that first visit, Anna underwent a face lift. She was so pleased with the results of the cosmetic surgery that she went on to have a tummy tuck as well as liposuction in those few areas that exercise just wouldn't budge.

Today Anna looks like the daughter of the woman who originally came to see me. And although her life is now rich and rewarding in every way, she deeply regrets having spent the time and trouble she could have saved had she not subjected her body to such early abuse.

Heredity

It's been said that you can choose your friends but not your relatives. And since genetic composition is the single most determining factor when it comes to assessing the rate at which your skin will age, one look at your family can either make your hopes for maintaining a youthful complexion soar or send them plummeting into the depths of despair.

If your senior-citizen parents are constantly being mistaken for your second-grader's mom and dad, rejoice! You've probably inherited a wonderful set of genes. If, on the other hand, your folks looked like senior citizens even when *you* were in the second grade, don't fret, for all is not lost. Your aging destiny is by no means cast in iron. Rather, it happens to be quite flexible and capable of change.

By carefully nurturing and protecting the support structure of your body's largest organ, you will be able to hold back the signs of time in your skin for years to come and, in so doing, will change the course of (your family's aging) history!

CHANGES TO EXPECT AFTER THIRTY DAYS

Combination skin will begin to normalize.

Surface facial wrinkles (such as those that commonly appear on the forehead, at the corners of the eyes, and between the nostrils and the sides of the mouth) will soften.

Feelings of lethargy will subside, replaced by a resurgence of energy.

Symptoms of insomnia will start to disappear; a general sense of well-being will be experienced.

The Second Thirty Days: Treating Special Problems

ACNE

This four-letter word spells trouble, a fact to which its millions of hapless victims can unequivocally attest; especially those who, like you, must treat the condition on two separate skintypes. Luckily, help has finally arrived! Through the pages of this chapter, you'll become privy to all of the information you'll need to put your problems with acne well behind you, once and for all.

My strategic defense plan begins with a little background material on your opponent, the world's most prevalent skin disease, and goes on to tell you what changes in lifestyle will do to improve your complexion, as well as what can be done about the problem *right now*!

The ''Family'' of Acne Lesions

Definitely not the sort to which you'd willingly extend an invitation, the members of this clan are the kind that tend to show up uninvited. Before we proceed any further, I'd like to make you aware of the wide variety of forms this most unwelcome intruder can take.

How Acne Begins

The skin is made up of three layers: the subcutaneous layer (or fatty tissue); the dermis (which houses the blood vessels, nerves, sweat glands, and follicles); and the epidermis (which covers the dermis and serves as the skin's "overcoat"). Running through the dermis is the connective tissue that, as its name implies, is the supporting structure of the dermis.

While the sweat glands have a direct opening to the surface of the skin, the oil (or sebaceous) glands are not quite as fortunate. The oil (or sebum) produced in these glands must find its way to the skin's surface via a follicle or pore, some of which contain hair. This is where the trouble can get its start. If the cells that line these follicles stick together instead of sloughing off (as they do under normal conditions), acne begins, and all forms of acne initiate in the very same manner. Now for a closer look:

MICROCOMEDO. This earliest form of acne plug is not visible to the naked eye. Nonetheless, microcomedones are insidious and can (and often do) lead to more serious things.

CLOSED COMEDO. This more advanced stage of the microcomedo is also called a whitehead. Since there is almost no opening at the surface, the closed comedo must never be squeezed; in so doing, you would only force its contents deeper into the skin and run the risk of scarring.

OPEN COMEDO. Better known as the blackhead, the open comedo is an acne plug with an opening at the surface. Because of this fact, the contents of the blackhead can usually be emptied by exerting gentle pressure on both of its sides. (Be sure to first steam skin for 15 minutes.) Always use your index fingers, making sure they're wrapped with tissues before you start. (*NOTE*: Never use a "comedo extractor" to remove blackheads, as these instruments can do serious damage to the surrounding skin.) If the material does not come out easily, don't force it! Follow with a dab of 3% hydrogen peroxide on a cotton ball.

Blackheads are not caused by dirt. Their darkish color comes partially from the oxidation of the sebum and partially from the skin's own pigment or melanin. Therefore, blackheads, cannot simply be washed away.

PUSTULE. A small red bump that peaks with a yellowish cap of pus is known as a pustule. It is basically a comedo that has ruptured, and when this happens, your body's white blood cells rush in like the infantry to fight the "foreign invaders," which include bacteria, oil, and dead cells.

You may try to drain this type of acne lesion and, if properly done, this process will greatly accelerate the healing of the area. First, make sure your hands are scrupulously clean. Next, sterilize a needle by holding it in the flame of a match for a few seconds. After the needle has cooled, puncture the pustule in the exact center of the yellowish cap. With index fingers wrapped in tissue, gently squeeze the sides of the lesion. Stop when the pus no longer comes out easily. If you force it, you will drive the material deeper into the skin and greatly increase the likelihood of permanent scarring. Now place a warm compress (a clean washcloth soaked in warm water will do) over the area for a few minutes and finish by pressing with a cotton ball dipped in rubbing alcohol.

Warm-water soaks can and should be repeated several times daily until the lesion has healed. The warm water increases the flow of blood to the area and hence, speeds up the healing process.

CYSTIC ACNE. If you have even one acne lesion that resembles a large boil or cyst, you should consider your condition severe and place yourself under the regular care of a qualified cosmetic dermatologist. If finances are worrying you, don't forget that most insurance companies cover acne treatments. Speak with your doctor.

My Step-by-step Method of Treatment

Mine is a multifactored approach to the treatment of acne. Although specific "routes" might vary slightly from patient to patient, in the end "all roads lead to Rome" (that is, clear skin).

STRESS. What better place to start than with a review of one of acne's primary aids and abetters—stress—and to reiterate the extremely detrimental effect it can have on skin. Have you ever experienced a breakout right before an unusually important event, perhaps your wedding or the start of a new job? It is the extra strain put on your emotions by these out-of-the-ordinary occasions that probably caused the blemishes to appear.

The chain of biological events that leads up to a breakout goes like this: Stress activates the hypothalamus gland, which in turn stimulates the pituitary gland. The pituitary sends a message to the adrenal gland indicating that a larger-than-normal number of male hormones (including androgen) should be released immediately. Androgen activates the oil glands to produce sebum, which can result in acne.

I've had cases in which excessive stress has caused patients to pick at blackheads so much that they've ended up creating serious cases of acne for themselves. And I've had one or two who didn't stop there but went on to pick at the scab, causing permanent scarring.

Since a certain amount of stress is simply part of life and is all right, the key to minimizing its adverse effects lies in the way we handle it. Learning to relax is the obvious solution, but very often this cannot be done by the individual acting alone. If, after thorough examination and testing, I feel that stress is at the root of the problem, I will suggest some form of psychological counseling to resolve the inner conflict.

EXERCISE. In more moderate cases of emotional stress (but ones that are clearly having an adverse effect on the skin), the addition of exercise to the daily routine may prove very beneficial. Not only does exercise stimulate the circulation and aid in the cleansing of the skin (by flushing out impurities through perspiration), it also reduces tension, thus improving one's mental outlook. And a positive outlook cannot be discounted when it comes to creating that "inner glow" so important to a beautiful complexion.

A few words of caution before you start, however. Since exercise does increase the activity of the sweat glands and a buildup of this perspiration can trap oils below the skin, you should always begin your regimen with a clean face and shower immediately after you're finished. Whenever possible, wear loose-fitting clothing while you work out, as chafing can aggravate acne on the back and chest. Finally, when selecting a form of exercise, it's wise to keep your choice in the "middle of the road" category— no marathons your first time out, please! Remember, too much of a good thing can sometimes be worse than nothing at all.

REST. Another important acne-combatant is adequate rest. Since the skin repairs and rejuvenates itself while we sleep, the importance of rest to a healthy complexion should be obvious. While needs tend to vary slightly from individual to individual, the stan-

My Ninety-Day Plan for Combination Skin

dard eight hours per night should suffice for most. What's that you say? You can't possibly devote eight whole hours a day to *just sleeping*? Well, as the old saying goes, if it's really important, you'll find the time for it, and the proper amount of sleep is vital if you want to see an improvement in the condition of your skin.

DIET. "You are what you eat": In my opinion, these are some of the truest words ever spoken. Although the exact correlation between diet and acne remains something of a debate among doctors, I prefer to err on the side of caution. In compliance with this philosophy, I ask that you closely adhere to my basic nutritional program, as well as add the following acne aggravators to your "to be avoided" list:

> All dairy products
>
> Beef (because of the hormones given the animals to fatten them)
>
> Cabbage, shellfish, spinach, artichokes, iodized salt, and kelp (because of the high iodine content of these foods)

VITAMINS AGAINST ACNE. For maximum effectiveness, please incorporate these acne-fighting supplements into your daily vitamin-therapy regime:

○ Vitamin A: 10,000 additional I.U.s (not to exceed 20,000 I.U.s under a doctor's supervision)
○ Zinc: an extra 50 mg.
○ Lysine (an amino acid): 500 mg.

Finally, by increasing your daily intake of wheat germ by 2 tablespoons (from 1 to 3), you'll be providing your body with the additional vitamin F it needs to slow down your skin's production of oil.

Guidelines to Non-prescription and Prescription Drugs that Go to Work Immediately

Since acne starts when the cells that line the follicle stick together, instead of sloughing off as they normally do, one way to prevent the disease is to stop the cells from sticking together in the first place.

Fortunately, this can be accomplished. All you need is the proper drying-peeling agent for your skin type and a bit of knowledge regarding its correct usage. Drying-peeling agents work because they contain chemicals that get down *into* the follicle, unlike cleansers and astringents, to peel apart the dead cells that are trying to stick together. These products must be used with great regularity and must be rubbed into the skin.

In order for you to derive maximum benefits from your drying-peeling agent, it is essential that you choose one specifically formulated for your type of skin.

The rating system that follows is a quick and easy way to determine your "range":

What is the texture of your skin?

If it's dry..score 0
If it's normal.......................................score 1
If it's oily ....score 2

What is the tone of your skin?

If it's light ....score 1
If it's medium.....................................score 2
If it's olive or dark ....score 3

What is the severity of your acne?

Fewer than 10 lesions on your face..............score 1
Between 10 and 25 lesions on your face ....score 2
Over 25 lesions on your face or
one large acne cyst................................score 3

If your total score falls between 1 and 3, you need a mild drying-peeling agent. Between 4 and 6 requires a moderate-strength medication. And a score of 7 or 8 demands a full-strength product.

The table below lists the most effective and readily available nonprescription products designed to serve the needs of those in each category.

Mild medications

Rezamid Acne Lotion
Fostex Medicated Cover-up
Clinique's Anti-Acne Formula

My Ninety-Day Plan for Combination Skin

Moderate-strength medications

Oxy 5*
Acne Aid Lotion
Loroxide Acne Lotion

Full-strength medications

Saligel
Stridex Maximum Strength Cream Treatment*
Clearasil Super Strength*

THE PROCESS. Start by applying the drying-peeling agent to your face once a day, after washing. To avoid unnecessary irritation of the skin, make sure the area is completely dry before applying the medication (waiting 15 or 20 minutes). Cover areas that are currently broken out, as well as those that have a tendency to be. *But do not cover your entire face!* The T-zone (forehead, nose, and chin) is usually the prime spot for acne, but be sure to avoid placing the medication around the eyes and corners of the mouth, as these areas are much too sensitive for this type of treatment.

IS THE MEDICATION WORKING? You will know if you observe the surface peeling of your skin. Although your skin will appear slightly dry, this drying and peeling action will in no way harm your skin, nor will it cause wrinkles. The only thing you might find discouraging after you start your treatment is the possible appearance of new acne lesions. Believe me when I say that these would have shown up sooner or later. They stem from existing microcomedones, and the peeling action simply brought them to

---

*These medications contain benzoyl peroxide—a very effective drying-peeling agent, but some people are allergic to it. Therefore, prior to beginning treatment with a product containing benzoyl peroxide, it is wise to do a patch test. Apply a small amount of the medication—about the size of a quarter—to a portion of the affected area for several consecutive days. If no irritation develops, you can proceed as planned. If, however, you are having an adverse reaction to the product, switch to a formula that contains one (or more) of the other nonprescription chemicals found in drying-peeling agents, including sulfur, resorcinol, and salicylic acid. (Spot coverups should never be confused with drying-peeling agents, for in order to qualify as such, the preparation must contain one or more of the aforementioned chemicals.)

Benzoyl peroxide is a bleaching agent. In order to avoid unwanted lightening of hair, clothes, and pillowcases, allow the product to dry completely before moving on. Finally, avoid products packaged with their own applicator, like Noxema's On-the-Spot. The constant touching and retouching of acne lesions with the same instrument makes one highly susceptible to reinfection. If you must carry medication such as this for the sake of convenience, also take along several disposable cotton-tipped swabs.

a head a little sooner than would have happened naturally. Remember, the important thing is to prevent new acne plugs from forming.

If your skin appears to be slightly reddened by the use of any acne medication, try applying one of the over-the-counter hydrocortizone cremes to the affected area: Cortaid or Lanacord, for example. This should be done after your drying-peeling agent has dried. The anti-inflammatory properties of these preparations should help to alleviate any minor irritation.

If your skin stops peeling or if your acne gets worse, you may have to alter your plan of action. Sometimes you need to strengthen your acne medication, which can be done in one of two ways: by increasing either the frequency of treatments or the strength of the drying-peeling agent. Never do both at the same time, thinking that if some is good, more is better. It isn't! You will know the change is working when peeling resumes. If the opposite is the case, that is, your medication seems to be too strong, take the reverse tack of decreasing either the frequency of treatments or the strength of the drying-peeling agent.

WINDING DOWN. After your acne has been under control for a period of four to eight weeks, you can begin a maintenance program. Once again, proceed with caution. Change one factor, one step at a time. Decrease the strength of the peeling agent or, if your acne was severe and you applied your medication twice a day, decrease it to just once. Remain at the lower level for at least two weeks before decreasing another step. Continue this downward progression until your face no longer peels. But if your acne flares up after you decrease your treatment, resume the level at which the condition was under control. Maintain that level until you once again feel confident enough to begin a "slow descent."

RETIN A (VITAMIN A ACID). One drying-peeling agent that requires a prescription is Retin A (tretinoin or retinoic acid, as it's sometimes known). Although the vast majority of acne sufferers will peel with an over-the-counter drying-peeling agent, there are some who will not. For these individuals, vitamin A acid can prove very effective in the clearing of the skin. But, as with any powerful drug, vitamin A acid is not without adverse side effects. Its usage may bring about intense surface peeling as well as extreme irritation in the skin of the patient who applies it too often or incorrectly. For this reason, I insist on close medical supervision of every individual engaged in this form of therapy.

Recently, Retin A has also proven an effective tool in the treatment of aging skin. While it is by no means a replacement for dermabrasion or the chemical peel, it will, through consistent usage, reverse some signs of photoaging (sun damage to the skin which causes premature aging) as well as minimize fine lines and wrinkles but must be used under medical supervision.

ACCUTANE. Another derivative of vitamin A used to treat very severe cases of cystic acne is the prescription drug accutane. Although touted by some as a wonder drug in treating difficult cases, my opinion is that dangers from the immediate (and unknown long-term) side effects brought on by the drug's usage, do outweigh its possible advantages. Of course, there is always the exception to the rule, but treatment with accutane is something I prescribe only as a last resort. Here are some of the reasons why: The most serious side effect produced by accutane is the documented fact that it can cause birth defects in unborn fetuses. Any woman of childbearing age who is contemplating using the drug should therefore submit to a pregnancy test and be carefully monitored by her doctor throughout the duration of treatment. In addition, accutane frequently causes excessively dry lips, nosebleeds, elevated lipid levels, pains and swelling in the joints, and occasional personality changes. Still, as it is sometimes the only thing that will bring really stubborn cases of acne under control, the afflicted individual is often willing to take the risks. Accutane is taken by mouth and the blood must be frequently monitored.

ANTIBIOTICS. The most widely prescribed antibiotic in the treatment of acne is tetracycline, which works by effecting the creation of fatty acids within the follicle. The most common side effect of taking tetracycline is the yeast infection it seems to produce in some women (a risk that can be minimized by adding two extra tablespoons of acidophilus to your daily "beauty cocktail"). Photosensitivity can also be a problem for some people, and tetracycline should be discontinued when going in the sun. If you are taking a multivitamin while on tetracycline, make sure it is a formula that does not contain iron, as that mineral blocks the body's absorption of the drug, and avoid milk products.

If tetracycline ceases to be effective in controlling a patient's acne, the doctor will often switch to erythromycin, an antibiotic that works in much the same way. Minocycline is a chemical derivative of tetracycline that has proven effective in some instances when plain tetracycline has failed. The side effects that accompany minocycline can be more severe than those experienced through the usage of tetracycline; one side effect is dizziness.

Sometimes such antibiotics as tetracycline, erythromycin, clindamycin, and lincomycin are used in topical applications with excellent results. The main advantage of a topical over a systemic medicine (one which enters the system) is in the reduced instances of side effects.

BIRTH CONTROL PILLS. When birth control pills were first introduced nearly thirty years ago, they contained very large doses of estrogen and almost always contributed to an improved complexion in acne sufferers. But since estrogens also generated many undesirable side effects, pharmaceutical manufacturers began introducing pills that were formulated with greatly reduced amounts of the hormone. Although these newer pills are easier for most women to take, they do not provide the same degree of relief from acne as did their predecessors. In fact, some formulations may even make the condition worse.

Birth control pills generally thought to help acne are Demulen, Enovid-E, Enovid-5, and Ovulen. Those that usually aggravate the disease include Norinyl, Norlestrin, Ortho-Novum, and Ovral. If you are currently taking one of the formulas believed to worsen acne, speak with your doctor about a possible change in your prescription. (Don't forget to take B-complex vitamins when taking birth control pills.)

INTRALESIONAL STEROID SHOTS. The times when I've felt a kinship to my fellow physicians the obstetricians are the times when I've had a model, actress, or other highly visible individual rushed into my office so that I might administer the "magical injection" that would deliver her to an impending photo shoot or TV commercial, blemish-free. (Fortunately, I've never been called out in the middle of the night for this!) These shots contain a dosage of corticosteroids that is injected directly into the acne lesion. Because the anti-inflammatory properties of cortisone rapidly shrink the blemish, it is usually gone within a couple of days. Occasional dimpling or depression in the skin can occur secondary to these intralesional steroid injections, but fortunately this dimpling is usually reversible and transitory.

Acne Scars Don't Have to Be Forever

I would be greatly remiss to conclude this section without mentioning the wide variety of cosmetic surgery procedures now available to aid in the correction of acne scars. Although I will explain each in the section devoted to cosmetic surgery, I can assure you that there is no need to wear the scars obtained in the heat of your battle with acne. Thanks to the many advances of modern technology, there are several very viable means for virtually eliminating them so that, in the end, "all that's left is the memory." Fortunately for acne sufferers, memories (unlike scars) do tend to fade completely with time!

COMBINATION SENSITIVE SKIN

The introduction of the "sensitivity" element to your skin's already dual personality adds yet another dimension to your role as caretaker. Still, if your complexion is to flourish (as it most assuredly can given the proper treatment), all of its needs must be met. To aid in your efforts, I'd like to provide the following very comforting suggestions:

> Be sure to wash bed linens, face cloths, towels, and any items of personal clothing in a mild, low-sudsing soap such as Ivory. Avoid at all costs regular detergents (which tend to leave a residue) as well as any other harsh products that may come in contact with your skin. If *total* avoidance is simply not possible (when cleaning, for example), protect yourself by wearing rubber gloves.

> Never use tissues (such as Kleenex) to remove makeup (or for any other purpose) on your face. They contain fine wood shavings that can easily scratch and irritate delicate skin. Pads of cotton are a much safer alternative.

> For facial cleansing, always be sure to use cloths made of 100 percent cotton. You can easily make these yourself by purchasing a package of cloth diapers and cutting them into squares of four. These cloths double as very convenient and soothing masks, if two pieces are alternately dipped in a basin of ice water to which a couple of drops of vinegar have been added. Allow one to rest

on your face until the chill has worn off, and then switch to the other piece. Keep doing this for 15 to 20 minutes to calm redness or irritation.

If your complexion is feeling particularly "touchy," avoid any sort of granular exfoliation (that is, one using sugar, salt, or cornmeal). Opt instead for this mask: Mash one papaya and apply to your entire face (and neck, if you wish). The enzyme in this fruit magically and *gently* "eats" the dead skin cells. You can wash them away in just 20 minutes (using tepid, then cool, water).

Use extra caution when bleaching or waxing facial hair, as this delicate area is very suseptible to problems. To be on the safe side, have it done professionally.

Last but not least, remember to handle your skin as little as possible. Don't rub your face vigorously, and above all, don't scratch it! If itching occurs, place an ice cube in a handkerchief and apply it to the area of itching for five or six seconds. The itching will stop!

SKIN DURING PREGNANCY AND MENOPAUSE

Pregnancy and the Combination Skin

Depending upon whether you tend to view your glass as half empty or half full, you'll probably find your skin during pregnancy to be either the best or the worst of both worlds. Being prepared for what's in store and ready to treat the duality of your complexion's needs is your single best defense against any potential problems. Here's what to expect:

The first half of your pregnancy will be accompanied by an increase in the production of the skin's oil; while this won't particularly benefit the oily sections of your face, it should prove a definite plus for the dry ones. During the second half, everything's in reverse, with the oily areas enjoying the distinct advantage.

A little extra effort on your part should be all that it takes for your skin to fare the whole experience very well. There's even a good chance it might actually *glow*!

Menopause

This is the time in your life when your two types of skin finally unite into one, as the oily areas begin to show signs of drying. For many, this has been a welcome relief and a day long awaited, when just one skincare regimen will suffice. Keeping your "new" complexion totally fit really involves only a little reprogramming. Remembering that your skincare responsibilities have been cut in half, however, shouldn't prove too tough an assignment!

One additional note: Because the symptoms of menopause can range from slightly annoying to downright hair-raising, some doctors have a tendency to overprescribe, (i.e. tranquilizers, sleeping pills, anti-anxiety/anti-depressants—all potentially habit-forming) in an effort to help their patients cope. Bear in mind that any medication can have an adverse effect on skin. Before taking it, always weigh the benefits against the potential side effects.

A brisk 30-minute walk each day can do wonders for your state of mind (not to mention body), so before submitting to chemical mood alteration (i.e. drugs), why not try the physical approach by making regular aerobic exercise (jogging, swimming, biking, or walking) an integral part of your life.

CHANGES TO EXPECT AFTER SIXTY DAYS

Your skin should be much less oily now, with signs of acne markedly decreased. The dryness should be significantly diminished as well.

Your eyes will begin to sparkle around this time, and the whites will be much clearer.

You should also be sleeping like a baby, right through the night!

The Third Thirty Days: Completing the Plan

BODY CARE

You'll find that the skin on your body derives the same positive effects from my anti-aging plan as the skin on your face.

Hands and Feet

Two areas are always a source of concern, regardless of one's skintype: the hands and the feet. For this reason, I'd like to provide you with an overview of preventative care for each.

Over the years, I've seen hundreds of women spend thousands of dollars in an effort to preserve the fresh-faced look of a girl of 25. But a problem occurs when the hands dangling out of their sleeves are decidedly those of a 50-year-old matron. For this reason, if a patient is undergoing a facial cosmetic surgery procedure I will frequently perform one on the hands as well.

Unless you are prepared to wear gloves every day for the rest of your life, don't let your hands "give you away." If you follow these simple suggestions, that will never happen:

Keep a bottle of moisturizer next to each sink in your home, and apply it to your hands after every washing.

Wear cotton-lined rubber gloves when submerging hands in water. A pair of plain, white (dyes are a potential irritant to the skin) cotton gloves may be worn under regular rubber gloves.

To prevent ugly brown spots from appearing, be sure to include your hands when applying daily sunscreen, one half hour before going in the sun. And when temperatures dictate the need for a coat, wear gloves as well.

Hands can also benefit from the masks you use on your face.

Keep your nails neatly manicured; they can be a distinct beauty asset, or a liability, if neglected.

Try massaging an antiperspirant into sweaty palms. This should help to alleviate any potential embarrassment. If you find it irritating, consult your doctor. There is a new process called ionophoresis that is effective.

Apply moisturizer to hands before going to bed, and, if they're feeling particularly rough and chapped, "lock it in" by wrapping them in a layer of Saran Wrap covered by a pair of white cotton gloves. The slight discomfort involved in this procedure is well worth the results it produces.

Our feet really take a beating each day, which is why nature provided us with an extra thick protective sole. However, if left unattended, the skin in this area becomes extremely thick, tough, and generally unattractive. Regularity of care is the key to prevent this from happening. If you follow these simple guidelines every day, your feet will keep you "walking on air" for the rest of your life:

At the end of the day, fill a small plastic basin with warm soapy water (you may prefer to use bath oil) and give your feet a good soak for at least 15 minutes (longer, if time permits).

Pat dry and go over any rough, calloused areas (such as heels) with a pumice stone. For stubborn callouses, try standing in an inch or two of bleach, which will have a softening effect. Pat dry after one minute and apply a good moisturizer.

Lavish with moisturizer and, one night a week (more if you wish), wrap your feet in Saran Wrap, as suggested for the hands, substituting white cotton socks for gloves.

It's also an excellent idea to prop your legs up with a couple of pillows and relax for 20 minutes each day. This reverses the pull of gravity your feet and legs are constantly exposed to and gives them a much-needed "breather."

Finally, be sure to change shoes, from high heels to low, very often. This relieves the calf muscles and keeps the Achilles tendon from becoming shortened.

Acne on the Back

Acne on the back is a frequent complaint. It seems to affect a wide cross-section of individuals of all skintypes. Here's the best way for everyone to bring it under control:

Always use a back brush and mild soap to properly cleanse the area during your daily shower or bath.

After the area is thoroughly dry, apply a slightly stronger drying-peeling agent (say, 10 percent benzoyl peroxide) than you'd use on your face. This suggestion is made because of the difficulty involved in reapplication of the product. (Thorough coverage of the area requires the aid of another person. If you live alone, just do the best that you can.)

Since it is not necessary to wash the area before the drying-peeling agent is applied, apply it once in the morning and once before retiring.

If the acne on your back is very severe, it may be necessary for you to add another bath or shower to your daily routine, at least until the condition has been brought under control. (Don't forget to remoisturize dry areas of the body immediately afterwards.)

Finally, if all of your attempts to bring the condition under control fail consult a dermatologist before scarring occurs. Some problems of this nature are very stubborn and will respond only to prescription-strength medication.

Warning: These Ingredients May Be Hazardous to the Health of Your Skin

The following potential irritants to combination skin, commonly found in treatment products, moisturizers and foundations are listed under the part of the face to which they apply.

Although they may not have troubled you as yet, skins do change. For this reason, always check the label of every new product before you buy it, especially if your skin is feeling particularly sensitive.

Oily Skin Irritants	*Dry Skin Irritants*
Detergents such as sodium lauryl & laureth-4	Camphor
Isopropyl myristate	Menthol
Isopropyl palmitate	Talc
Butyl stearate	Alcohol
Isostearyl neopentanoate	Magnesium aluminum Silicate
Cetyl oleate	Detergent-based cleansers
Octyl palmitate	Fragrance
Isocetyl stearate	
Lanolin	
Fragrance	
Preservatives	

SUN SPECIFICS

Aging's first lieutenant in the field, the sun is beauty's greatest natural enemy. Although total avoidance is your only secure defense, it would be difficult to imagine a life lived entirely on the "inside." In lieu of that approach, here are some of the most effective ways I've found to minimize the effects of the sun:

Get into the sunscreen habit. Apply one with an SPF of at least 15 every morning, alone or under makeup, one half hour before going in the sun. (With SPF 15 protection, the skin can tolerate the sun 15 times longer than without a protective product. With SPF 4, 4 times longer, etc.) I believe sunscreen of SPF 15 or 20 is about the most effective you can get today. More than that is wishful thinking.

To protect areas that are among the first to show signs of aging, always include hands and neck in your sunblock coverage.

Because the skin on your lips contains very little melanin, this area requires SPF protection of its own. Make sure it gets it by regularly using one of the "lip blocks" on the market, either alone or under your lipstick. (By the way, the brighter the shade, the better the protection.) Remember to reapply frequently whenever you're out in the sun, and always after eating or drinking.

Don't forget your sunglasses. Wear them twelve months of the year! Best are the wraparound kind and ones that indicate their UV (Ultra Violet) protection. To further shield this delicate area, use one of the sunblocks created specifically for use around eyes.

Hats (especially the wide-brimmed variety) are always in style when it comes to spending a day in the sun.

Avoid taking PABA by mouth. Taken orally, it frequently incites a negative reaction in the skin.

Don't believe the ads: Sun beds and tanning booths are every bit as detrimental to skin as the real thing.

All of the following can make you extra sensitive to sun. If you must be in it, avoid them:

Many medications, including antibiotics, birth control pills, diuretics, and tranquilizers. Check with your doctor to see if anything else you might be taking applies.

Germicidal soaps and antiseptics that contain hexachlorophene and bithionol.

Any product that's alcohol based, such as astringent, perfume, after-shave, and cologne.

Excessive amounts of vitamins A and C. (More than 20,000 I.U.s of vitamin A a day or more than 2,000 mgs. of vitamin C a day.)

Remember: *Be afraid of your own shadow*! It's there to remind you that the sun's damaging rays are lurking close by.

CHANGES TO EXPECT AFTER NINETY DAYS

Combination skin should have completely normalized by now, with both dry and oily areas dramatically less so.

Surface facial wrinkles will have all but disappeared, making you look substantially younger than you did three short months ago.

The skin on the backs of your hands will have tightened, significantly, making them much more youthful in appearance.

Your energy level will have peaked. You'll feel on top of the world and never more alert.

My Ninety-Day [   ] Plan for Dry Skin

Although, in general, dry skin fares the best early in life, things start to decline rapidly when Father Time enters the picture. Dry skin is the most vulnerable to time's earliest advances and hence is almost always the first to reveal the visible signs of aging.

Fortunately, there is a way around all of this—a detour of sorts. Through the guidelines set forth in my plan, you'll experience a new level of moisture in your skin and a reversal of aging you would never have believed possible! So let's get started—after all, there's no time to waste!

With a family history of autoimmune diseases, Cynthia always knew her chances for acquiring one of them were strong. Unfortunately, her fear became a reality, and sooner than she might have expected.

A professional ballerina for seven years, Cynthia's career was brought to a halt when she was awakened one morning by severe pain and swelling in both ankles. An immediate consultation with a specialist in the field of rheumatology confirmed her suspicion: She was suffering from acute rheumatoid arthritis.

Over the next five years, Cynthia underwent extensive treatments with powerful anti-inflammatory drugs, including steroids. While they did aid in keeping the symptoms of her disease under control, they also left her complexion unbearably dry and lackluster. She came to me for help.

I immediately started her on a regime of advanced vitamin therapy (built around the core of my dry-skin formula), which I augmented to include: 1 gm. of alfalfa, three times a day; 2 tablets of yucca extract, twice daily (both natural anti-inflammatory agents); 2,000 additional mgs. of vitamin C (to counter the depletion in her system caused by the excessive amounts of aspirin she'd been advised to take); and extra vitamin B-complex. I suggested that she also incorporate into her plan daily supplements of coenzyme Q-10 (CoQ-10) and germanium, two organically derived substances, available at health food stores, that are believed to boost the immune system.

Armed with an outline of my basic anti-aging nutritional program for dry skin, as well as my regime for its most effective daily care (stressing frequent warm herbal masks), she left the office vowing to give the natural approach a fair try.

I'm elated to report that, while I'm not usually a believer in miracles, I certainly witnessed one in Cynthia. In just eleven months, her skin was soft, supple, and radiant with the glow of good health. Filled with a renewed sense of vitality, she relayed to me the most exciting and remarkable news of all: Her arthritis was in complete remission! Although her rheumatologist could offer no specific explanation for the phenomenon, he had to agree she was clearly on the right track and encouraged her to continue with her vitamin and nutrition therapies.

That was almost three years ago. Cynthia still lives by my approach and remains virtually arthritis free. She says she looks and feels better than she did ten years ago, and is even considering a return to the world of dance, this time in a teaching capacity.

An inspiration to all who know her, Cynthia exudes the confidence of one who has triumphed over seemingly insurmountable odds, for, by not succumbing to destiny's threat, she believes she has truly slain the Goliath of her family legacy.

By the time Claire G. came in for her first visit, she needed no reminder of the toll years of nutritional self-neglect had taken on her. She faced it in the mirror each day.

Admittedly a "weight-loss junkie," Claire's frequent and often inadequate diets had left her body vitamin starved. Of particular concern were the rough and scaly patches on her skin (evidence of a marked deficiency in vitamin A).

To make matters worse, the emotional upheaval of a recent divorce (and subsequent medical treatment for the depression surrounding it) had turned her already-dry complexion parched and dull. She believed (correctly) that the whole ordeal had also contributed to a substantial loss of her hair.

An attorney, she felt overworked at her job, but—with partnership in sight—was compelled to perform at her peak. Not surprisingly, she was chronically fatigued and appeared visibly shaken as she told me of her plight.

Assuring her things were bound to improve, I got her started by outlining a more natural system for total body healing and sustained good health. Relying on my basic anti-aging nutritional and vitamin therapies for the dry-skinned individual, I customized her specific plan with additions of the following: 100 mcg. of biotin (vitamin H); 500 mg. of cysteine (for hair and skin); two B-complex supplements; 1,000 mg. of vitamin C (both for stress); and 25,000 I.U.s of beta carotene (to correct her deficiency in vitamin A). (These dosages were over and above the ones already indicated on her basic plan.) Finally, I prescribed a 1 percent solution of minoxidil (for direct application to the scalp) to aid in the regrowth of her thinning hair. (This drug, available by prescription only, was originally developed as an antihypertensive. It has recently been found effective in treating certain cases of early male-pattern baldness. Minoxidil therapy should never be undertaken without the supervision of a doctor.)

Claire promised to take better care of herself, through strict adherence to all facets of my plan. With a wish for good luck, I sent her on her way.

Claire's loyalty most assuredly paid off. In only six months, she was a changed person. Her skin glowed (for the first time in her life) with an aura of good health, and a regrowth of hair was clearly visible. She was absolutely thrilled by the fact that my nutritional regime had afforded her an effortless as well as healthful weight loss (one that she'd maintained) and, no longer feeling the need, she had stopped the medications prescribed for her bouts with anxiety.

The last time we spoke, Claire informed me she had just been made partner at the Wall Street law firm where she'd "slaved" as an associate for close to eight years. Her only regret, she conceded, was that she had to "bottom out" before seeking the help that had so dramatically improved her life.

These are only two of the hundreds of examples of lives that have literally been turned around, thanks to my revolutionary

My Ninety-Day Plan for Dry Skin

approach to naturally beautiful skin. And the next one can be yours!

Everything you need to declare a personal "war on time" is contained in the pages of this section. For the sake of the yet-to-be-discovered beauty in you, why not get started today?

The First Thirty Days: De-aging the Skin

DAILY CARE

Your personal care, every day, is the most important element in maintaining beautiful, young-looking skin; without a meticulously cared-for complexion, one can never hope to fulfill one's true beauty potential. With this in mind, I've developed the following "natural alternatives" to more traditional treatment products. Created especially for use on dry skin, the formulas are all very easy to prepare, inexpensive, and extremely effective. Once you've tried them and seen for yourself the difference they can make, I'm certain you'll never use another thing on your face.

Here is your program of daily care.

Morning

STEP 1: CLEANSING. To awaken, dry skin usually requires no more than a few splashes of warm, followed by cool, water. For the sake of convenience, try misting the face with a noncarbonated mineral water (a plant mister is fine for this purpose).

STEP 2: NOURISHING. While skin is still damp, lock in moisture by applying one of the three nourishing alternatives described below. Remember to lavish on face and neck (both front and back).

Either: A thin layer of margarine (the kind sold in health food stores) that contains no artificial colorings, flavorings, or preservatives. (Amazingly, when topically applied, the margarine sinks right into skin, leaving no greasy residue.)

Or: A light application of mayonnaise. To insure its quality, try making it yourself, using the following recipe:

> To 1 slightly beaten egg yolk, add a cup of olive oil, 1 teaspoon at a time. When the mixture starts to thicken, whisk in a teaspoon of fresh lemon juice, and voilà—the "makings" of smooth skin! Mayonnaise can be stored for four or five days in a tightly closed jar and kept in a refrigerator. Be sure to restir before each usage.

Or: If mayonnaise or margarine don't appeal to you, a light application of olive or any cold-pressed oil is also good.

Evening

STEP 1: MAKEUP REMOVAL. Any thin, natural, cold-pressed oil may be used for this purpose, with avocado, olive, and safflower oils all registering as popular choices. Simply massage oil lightly over the face and throat, removing it with pads of damp cotton. Repeat until the last traces of oil and makeup have disappeared.

STEP 2: CLEANSING. Apply 2 or 3 tablespoons of plain, natural yogurt (very soothing) to damp skin, and massage well over entire face and throat area. Follow with 20 splashes of tepid water to insure that no residue remains on skin.

STEP 3: EXFOLIATING. Necessary for removing the dead cell accumulation so common to dry skin, this procedure, when performed on a regular basis, has proven very effective in the removal of such flaky buildup, which also impedes your moisturizer's "power of penetration." Simply mix a small amount of yellow cornmeal (enough to make a thin paste) with water, and gently massage the mixture over the face and throat with fingertips to loosen debris from the surface of pores. Finish with a warm water rinse, followed by a cool splash.

If your skin is extremely dry and easily irritated, try this exfoliating trick: Mash 1 papaya, which contains an enzyme that literally eats dead skin debris, and apply it to the face. Relax for 20 minutes before removing the mixture in the manner described above.

STEP 4: TONING. Stir ½ teaspoon apple cider vinegar into 8 ounces of water. Apply to face and throat with pads of dampened cotton in an upward, sweeping motion. Besides being a very efficient toner, this preparation will restore the acid balance (or normal pH) to skin.

As an alternative, mix 3½ ounces each of strongly brewed rose hips tea and chamomile tea with 1 ounce of lemon juice. Shake until blended and apply in a similar manner.

MASKS. To enhance the effects of any mask, gently steam your face before applying. Simply toss a few bags of chamomile tea into a pot of boiling water, remove from the stove, and drape a towel over your head in a tentlike fashion to capture the steam.

The masks you can make yourself are every bit as varied and effective as those you can buy. (I believe they are more so.) Always apply after cleansing, ideally once or twice a week. Here are some of the best I've found for the treatment of dry skin. Masks should be made fresh before every application.

> **For a super (yet nondrying) peel.** Fold ½ cup dry-grind oatmeal into a whipped whole egg and lightly massage mixture into face (neck and hands, too!) Let remain on skin for 20 minutes before removing with a clean damp cloth or a warm water splash.

> **For a complete facial therapy.** Follow with a healing herbal mask. Mix 2 tablespoons avocado oil with a like amount of wheat germ oil and heat, over low flame, in top of double boiler. When it tests (on the skin of your forearm) as comfortably warm (never too hot), apply to face and neck, and allow to stand for 15 to 20 minutes.

> **To improve skintone.** Place 1 drop of lemon juice into 3 tablespoons honey and spread over the skin. Gently tap the treatment area for 3 to 5 minutes, as this motion draws blood to the skin's surface, enabling it to purify itself.

TOPICAL TREATMENTS AND WHY THEY WORK SO WELL

Apple cider vinegar. Restores skin to proper pH (acid/alkaline) balance.

Lemon. Rich in vitamin C, potassium, and iron, it gives tone to the skin and acts as a mild bleach.

Nail-polish remover. When applied with cotton-tipped swab to *individual blemishes only*, the acetone it contains rapidly dries up the lesions, thus accelerating the healing process.

Oatmeal or Wheatena. Gently exfoliates and deep-cleanses the skin. It also soothes irritations.

Vodka. As a very pure form of alcohol, it is a very effective astringent for tightening pores.

White sugar. An extremely efficient skin exfoliant, with the added advantage of having a slightly antibacterial effect on the complexion.

Yogurt. Cleanses and soothes the skin: reduces visible signs of irritation.

Milk of magnesia. Has a very healing effect on acne. Since it is slightly drying to the skin, its usage should be confined to individual lesions only.

To retexturize skin. Steep a handful of rosemary in 4 ounces of boiling water for 20 minutes. Strain and cool. Add 2 egg whites and 2 tablespoons powdered milk, and mix well. Allow mask to dry on skin for 20 minutes, while resting. Remove with damp clean cloth, or a warm water splash.

For a soothing treat. Mix 1 tablespoon wheat germ oil with ½ mashed avocado. Apply and relax, as it nourishes your skin, for 20 minutes or longer. The vitamin E in the avocado is a real delicacy for your dry complexion. Indulge! Remove with warm damp cloth or a warm water splash.

To correct dry patches. Puree 1 peeled banana with 1 tablespoon of olive oil. Allow to remain on extra dry, scaly patches for 20 to 30 minutes. Remove with damp clean cloth or a warm water splash.

TO HYDRATE THE SKIN. To dehydrate already dry skin is to add insult to injury. To make sure this never happens to yours, practice the following ''hydration ritual'' as frequently as possible:

Apply predigested liquid protein with soluable collagen (the kind once used, rather dangerously, for dieting and still available at most health food stores). The moisture should be evenly spread over face and neck. (A wooden tongue depressor—available at most drug stores—may be used for this purpose.) Allow to dry and remain on skin for 1 or 2 hours, lightly spritzing the area with water at 15 to 20 minute intervals. Rinse well after allotted time has passed. The hydrating effect this has on skin seems to last for several days following application.

TO REDUCE UNDER-EYE SWELLING AND BAGS. Cut a raw fig in half and place a section over each eye. Relax for 15 to 20 minutes. Or try placing 2 slices from inside an Idaho potato over eyes for the same amount of time.

NUTRITION AND VITAMIN THERAPY
Building Strength from Within

Have you ever heard anyone ask, ''Is it surgery or sardines?'' as they pondered the reason for someone's particularly young, attractive appearance? While the answer to that query could be a combination of the two, you may not be aware of the significant role the lowly sardine can play in maintaining beautiful skin.

On the anti-aging nutritional team, the sardine could easily be voted most valuable player, for this humble fish has the profound distinction of being the only food to double its already high content of RNA (ribonucleic acid) and DNA (deoxyribonucleic acid) while in the can.

RNA and DNA are the ''stuff cells are made of.'' And cells—by the millions—are the things that make up our bodies, each with a lifespan of approximately two years. Before the cell dies, it reproduces itself on orders given by a commander-in-chief (DNA) and carried out by a messenger (RNA). In theory, therefore, we should look the same today as we did ten or fifteen years ago. But unfortunately, as with most theories, this one has holes in it.

Because of a variety of external factors beyond our control, the cell goes through some deterioration with each successive reproduction, causing an alteration in its shape. The further away it moves from its original blueprint, the more visibly we show signs of aging.

Interestingly and very encouragingly, however, the matter is not entirely out of our hands. Work pioneered by the late Benjamin Frank, M.D. demonstrated that if we keep our bodies well supplied with external sources of the nucleic acids (like sardines), we can rejuvenate the cells to the point where the aging process is drastically retarded or even reversed. In addition, we will be contributing to an overall improvement in appearance as well as to a general sense of well-being. And therein lies the basis for my anti-aging nutritional plan, which will, if carefully followed, change much more than simply the way you eat.

So if you're ready to start feeling stronger, thinking more clearly, aging more slowly, and looking much, much better, I invite you to proceed to the specifics of the plan.

*My Anti-aging Nutritional Plan**

Four days per week, have a 3- or 4-ounce can of sardines.

Three other days per week, have one of the following: a serving of salmon, tuna, sole, bluefish, scrod, or monkfish.

Once or twice a week, have a serving of liver (chicken liver is best).

Have 2 or 3 eggs each week, if your cholesterol level is not elevated. (If there's a question, check with your doctor.)

Everyday, include 1 serving of fresh pineapple or papaya, in addition to 1 serving of any other fresh fruit.

Twice a week, have a serving of lentils, peas, lima beans, or soybeans, as well as a serving of avocado.

*If you are currently under a physician's care, check with your doctor before embarking on this or any other specialized nutritional program.

Each day, have a salad prepared with some or all of the following ingredients: spinach, mushrooms, onions, asparagus, radishes, celery, scallions, beets, carrots, and broccoli.

Have 1 tablespoon each of bran, wheat germ, brewer's yeast, and lecithin granules daily.

Two or three times per week, have a serving of oatmeal.

Include in your daily beverage intake all of the following: 1 glass of fruit or vegetable juice, 2 glasses of skimmed milk, and 6 to 8 glasses (8 oz.) of pure (preferably bottled) water.

Have oat bran muffins for breakfast frequently. It lowers cholesterol and is great for fiber.

Finally, to detoxify your system and keep it running smoothly, enjoy this daily "beauty cocktail": Mix 3 tablespoons liquid acidophilus (friendly bacteria) and 1 tablespoon lactose into an 8-ounce glass of water, and drink to good health . . . yours! (Both acidophilus and lactose can be found in your local health food stores.)

If you stick strictly to this diet—with no additions—you'll lose weight. If weight is not a problem for you, the aforementioned foods may be incorporated into your regular diet, provided it does not include any of the following foods, which must be *avoided at all costs*:

Anything containing white flour or sugar; for sweetening, small amounts of honey or blackstrap molasses make healthy alternatives.

Alcoholic beverages; try Perrier and lemon or lime instead.

Red meat; dark poultry meat is all right.

Salt; garlic can be used in many instances as a substitute.

Fats; cold-pressed oils, such as safflower, are permitted in moderation.

Products containing caffeine; herbal teas are fine.

Bringing on the Reinforcements

Each day, include the following vitamin and mineral supplements in your diet:

One high-potency multivitamin containing chelated minerals after breakfast. ("Chelated" is your key to no stomach upset from certain supplements. Look for it on labels.)

One RNA/DNA tablet (125 mg.) after lunch. (Not to exceed daily intake of 150 mg.—including multivitamin)

Two high-potency B-complex vitamin tablets, one after breakfast and one after lunch. (Not to exceed total daily intake including multivitamin—of 100 mg. of each of the following: Vit. B-1, Vit. B-2, Vit. B-6, Vit. D, and 100 mcg. of Vit. B-12, 400 mcg. of folic acid, and 300 mcg. of Biotin.)

Two vitamin C tablets with bioflavinoids (500 mg. each), one after eating. (Not to exceed total daily intake—including multivitamin—of 1,000 mg. Higher doses may cause stomach upset.)

Vitamin E (800 I.U.s, dry form), once a day after breakfast. (Not to exceed total daily intake—including multivitamin—of 800 I.U.s.)

Selenium (100 mcg.) once a day, taken in conjunction with vitamin E. (Not to exceed intake of 100 mcg.—including multivitamin)

Vitamin A (10,000 I.U.s) daily after lunch. (Not to exceed total daily intake—including multivitamins—of 20,000 I.U.s)

Chelated zinc (50 mg.) daily after breakfast. (Not to exceed intake of 100 mg—including multivitamin per day)

Cysteine, an amino acid (500 mg.), midafternoon with a glass of either orange or grapefruit juice. (Not to exceed intake of 500 mg. daily—including multivitamin)

If this seems like a lot to swallow, imagine what a bitter pill it would be to discover, too late, that many of your blemishes, lines, and wrinkles were preventable.

Putting the Plan into Action for You

What follows is an outline of a typical day on my anti-aging nutritional plan.

BREAKFAST

High-energy shake made with:

    8 ounces skim milk
    ½ cup fresh raspberries
    1 tablespoon each, brewer's yeast and lecithin granules
    Honey, to taste
    2–3 ice cubes (for thickness)
    Mix on high speed in blender until frothy.

Bowl of cooked oatmeal sprinkled with 1 tablespoon each of bran and wheat germ.

Herbal tea

After breakfast, the following supplements:

    1 high-potency multivitamin/multimineral
    1 vitamin B-complex tablet
    500 mg. vitamin C with bioflavinoids
    800 I.U.s vitamin E (dry form)
    100 mcg. selenium
    50 mcg. chelated zinc

SUGGESTED FOODS AND HOW THEY BENEFIT YOUR SYSTEM

Sardines. Highest single source of nucleic acids (RNA/DNA). The only food to double such content while in the can.

Oatmeal or Wheatena. Also a good source of RNA/DNA, as well as natural fiber. When paired with bran, has been shown to be effective in reducing levels of cholesterol.

Papaya. Contains valuable digestive properties as well as valuable nutrients.

Lentils. Excellent alternate source of protein; also rich in nucleic acid.

Lecithin. Used in the making of chocolate to keep it from hardening before its time; has a similar effect on one's arteries. Also, an important moisture-binding agent.

Yogurt. Furnishes useful bacteria that keep the intestines clean by countering toxic substances.

The reason for one firm "no no"—alcohol. Especially when taken with meals, it tends to raise levels of uric acid, the very thing the diet strives to prevent by emphasizing fluids.

LUNCH

Cup of borscht (beet soup, served hot or cold)

Large spinach salad (including mushrooms, onions, and a hard-boiled egg), topped with a tablespoon each of safflower oil and red-wine vinegar

Serving of fresh pineapple

Perrier and lime

After lunch, these supplements:

125 mg. RNA/DNA tablet
10,000 I.U.s vitamin A
1 vitamin B-complex tablet

MIDAFTERNOON

500 mg. cysteine with 4 ounces of grapefruit juice

DINNER

½ avocado with lemon

Bouillabaisse (Mixed-seafood stew)

Small green salad

Dish of strawberries (fresh)

Herbal tea

After dinner, this supplement:

500 mg. vitamin C with bioflavinoids

If weight is not a problem for you, the aforementioned meals may be augmented as you wish, excluding, of course, the foods on the "to be avoided" roster.

Last, but not least, be creative! And remember to view each and every dining experience as the wonderfully rejuvenating treat for your skin that it is.

Sardine "Surprises"

Sardines are an amazingly versatile (not to mention incredibly healthy) food that should be eaten often. Here are a few innovative ways to maximize their appeal:

Peppers Stuffed with Sardines

2 large green peppers
3½ oz. can sardines (water packed), chopped
1 cup cooked rice
1½ medium-sized onion, minced
½ cup tomato sauce
1 egg
Salt and pepper

With a paring knife, cut a circle around the stem of each pepper. Pull out the stems, and, with a fork or teaspoon, scrape away as many of the seeds from the hollow as you can. Rinse them out with cold water.

Mix the sardines with the rice, the onion, and the tomato sauce. Beat the egg and add this along with approximately ½ teaspoon of salt and a dash of pepper.

Put this mixture into the hollow peppers, and bake for about 20 minutes at 350° F.

Sardines with Gouda Cheese

This makes a superb easy-to-cook main dish for two.

2 3½-ounce cans sardines
1 pound spinach
1½ cup skimmed milk

3 tablespoons corn oil margarine
3 tablespoons flour
2 teaspoons Worcestershire sauce
¾ cup crumbled Gouda cheese

Drain the sardines into a large frying pan, and set the sardines aside.

Wash the spinach and tear it into bite-sized pieces. Heat the sardine oil and pile spinach onto it. Cover and cook over low heat for 5 minutes, until the margarine melts.

While the spinach is cooking put 1 cup of the skimmed milk into a saucepan with the margarine. Heat over very low heat until the margarine melts.

Mix the flour into the rest of the skimmed milk, and pour the mixture slowly into the heating milk while stirring. Add the Worcestershire sauce, and all but 3 tablespoons of the cheese. Continue stirring until cheese melts, making sure the mixture does not boil.

Put the cooked spinach into a greased baking dish. Then place the sardines on top of the spinach and the cheese sauce on top of everything. Sprinkle the rest of the cheese on this, and bake at 400° F until the cheese melts (about 10 minutes).

A Canapé

Very lightly toast 2 slices of white bread. Cut each slice into 4 pieces. Mash 3½ ounces of sardines with a fork and spread over the bread pieces. Top with a few shavings of Swiss cheese and bake at 350°, until the cheese melts.

COMBATING THE SABOTEURS OF YOUNG SKIN

The time bandits that fall into this category have been guilty of bringing on an "early frost" in more cases than I'd care to mention, so let's examine the ways in which each of them contribute to the skin's demise and what can be done to minimize the damage.

For starters, you have an extremely powerful ally in your running battle with time, running right out of your kitchen and bathroom faucets! That's right, good old H_2O can be your single best defense when it comes to beating the clock, so be sure to take full advantage. Since, however, one can never be sure of the quality of tap water, it's best to either install a charcoal filter or drink the bottled variety.

The following are some of water's many and varied uses. I strongly suggest you immediately incorporate each of them into your daily life:

> Increase your consumption of the liquid by having at least 1 quart each day. This will aid in the removal of toxins from your system, which in turn will prevent them from having a negative impact on your skin (especially important for clearing a blemished complexion). Keep a pitcher of chilled water in the refrigerator at all times. For a refreshing and slightly tangy change of pace, try adding a few slices of fresh lemon to the container before storing.

> If you haven't done so already, purchase a humidifier and keep it going in your bedroom while you sleep. It's a small investment that will pay big dividends in moisture restored to your skin. If you rely on a humidifier instead of additional lubricant to keep your complexion moist at night, you'll substantially lessen the risk of "over-nourishing" your skin. (Be sure to change the water daily.)

> When washing your face, always rinse with twenty splashes of tepid water. Rehydrate often throughout the day by "spritzing" the area with one of the mineral waters (Evian, for example) sold in an aerosol can. This is especially important when traveling by air, as the pressurized cabins are extremely drying to skin. For the same reason, make your cocktails Perrier or another bottled water instead of alcohol.

Sun

Because of the overwhelmingly negative impact the sun has on skin, I've devoted an entire section to it ("Sun specifics" in "The Third Thirty Days: Completing the Plan") for your enlightenment. Precautions should be taken at all times—no matter what the weather. But if you're planning a vacation to the tropics where sun exposure is imminent, extra caution should be taken.

Exposure

When it comes to the aging effects of the elements (wind, heat, cold), total avoidance is your best defense. Unfortunately, from the day you leave the hospital in your mother's arms, this is a virtually impossible task, so the next best thing is to always take the proper precautions. Be sure to apply a sunscreen with an SPF of at least 15 every morning (alone or under make-up); wear sunglasses all year round whenever you're exposed to the sun, regardless of the temperature; wear protective clothing (i.e. heat reflecting in the summer and insulated in the winter, including hats and gloves.)

When I speak of "the elements," you probably think this refers only to the ones we're exposed to out of doors. On the contrary, the seasonal accommodations we make indoors (central heating and air conditioning) are every bit as detrimental to the health of your skin as their fresh-air counterparts. (Remember, it's water, not oil, that keeps skin moist.) Therefore, environmental protection on both fronts is definitely in order. Don't forget the humidifier. This is especially important in winter. Also keep plants around. They're good for your skin.

Make certain your skincare routine changes whenever your wardrobe does. Winter's cold and gusty winds are far more drying to skin than summer's heat and humidity, so be certain to cleanse, tone, and moisturize accordingly.

Facial Stress

Squinting, sneering, scowling, pursing the lips, knitting the brow—all common, everyday habits that happen to be major contributing factors to a condition known as facial stress: the self-inflicted damage done to facial muscles through chronic grimacing and general fatigue.

Although these reflexes are in some cases deeply ingrained in the mannerisms of an individual, for most people an awareness of their existence is usually all it takes to arrest the problem.

A patient once came to see me requesting collagen injections in the furrows of her brow. After noting the wrinkle-free appearance of the rest of her face, I advised that she might unconsciously be causing or aggravating the lines. To verify this fact, I suggested that she place a mirror on her desk at work and one near her telephone at home.

By setting up a "wrinkle watch" in this manner, she became aware that she was fervently knitting her brow during every telephone conversation. Once the collagen injections had corrected the problem, I suggested she might avoid a recurrence by placing small strips of hair-setting tape over the susceptible areas while at home. The slight tightening effect this produced at every twist and turn served as a more than sufficient deterrent whenever her face decided to "go into motion."

The same technique can be applied to any area of the face that is noticeably more lined than the rest. By closely observing the bad habits you probably didn't even realize you had, you can usually put a stop to them and, hence, the damage that results.

Now that you know how to stop these facial distortions "in their tracks" (or hopefully before they've left any permanent ones on your face), here are some other ways they get their start:

> Smoking is a double offender. Inhaling entails the pursing of the lips, while exhaling causes the eyes to squint (a reaction of self-defense to prevent the smoke from entering). In addition, smoking depletes the body's supply of Vitamin C, vital for its production of collagen.

> Another frequent cause of squinting is poor vision. To avoid this problem, see your ophthalmologist regularly and keep your prescription for corrective lenses up to date.

> Making a concerted effort to get all the sleep you need (for most this means the standard eight hours per night) can be a great beauty boon, as a lack of sleep really does "show on your face." Skin cells repair and rejuvenate themselves during periods of slumber, so opt for nine hours whenever possible.

> Try training yourself to sleep on your back (or at least start the night out in that position). It just might help put an end to the formation of lines and wrinkles that are a result of your face pressing against the pillow night after night. (Satin-cased pillows are best, by the way.)

The Use and Abuse of Alcohol

In addition to dehydrating the system and depleting the body's supply of the B vitamins, long-term consumption of alcohol can lead to dilation of the blood vessels. Eventually this can result in a condition known as rosacea, which gives the nose a red, blotchy, bulbous appearance. And let's face it, no matter how popular a nostalgia craze becomes, you might long for Cleopatra's eyes and adore Mona Lisa's smile, but one look no one will ever want is that of W. C. Fields's nose (the most famous case of rosacea)! If you're not already "on the wagon," for your skin's sake please climb aboard.

Emotional Stress

It flushes with embarrassment and rage, and it blanches with fear. There's no doubt about it, your skin truly is your body's emotional barometer.

If you have any doubt about just how aging chronic stress can be, compare two photographs of almost any official elected to high public office: one taken upon entering, the other on leaving the job. Such an image is worth more than a thousand words of warning. I treat many of these individuals, and, as a group, they challenge my skills for holding time at bay more than any other.

Since, however, stress is a fact of life that can never be completely eliminated, we must find a way (anything from self-hypnosis to psychotherapy) of handling it. The important thing is to discover a relaxation technique that works for you and to practice it regularly.

Lack of Exercise

Besides being a great source of stress relief (especially the aerobic variety), exercise flushes impurities out of the system through perspiration, improves circulation by carrying increased oxygen to cells, and firms and tones the muscles. It should therefore be apparent to even the greatest skeptic, that exercise plays a vital role in postponing the visible signs of aging. Exercise is the body's fountain of youth.

If you're not currently engaged in a regular sport—whether it be walking, jogging, swimming, or bicycling—find an activity you enjoy, start slowly, and build up the pace. Three times a week for at least one half hour is essential for cardio-pulmonary function as well as terrific skin. The vast improvement in the way you look and feel will serve as more than sufficient incentive for continuing.

In addition, you can reverse the pull of gravity, to a certain extent, by standing on your head or lying on a slantboard with your feet elevated for ten minutes each day. (Any 6- to 8-foot-long plank of wood—at least 10 inches wide—can be used.) Along with increasing the flow of blood to the dermis (creating a glow in the complexion), this action is an excellent energizer. (*A word of warning*: this position can cause extra pressure on the eyes. For those who are predisposed to conditions such as glaucoma, it could create or aggravate a problem. It is therefore best to check with your doctor before beginning).

Rapid and Frequent Changes in Weight

If you abuse your body by subjecting it to the "yo-yo" dieting syndrome, you are doing your skin more of a disservice than if you remained consistently overweight. The skin's elasticity is by no means "snap-proof," and if the body's supply of fat is constantly being depleted and restored, its resiliency simply wears out. Left with improper support, the irreversibly stretched skin can be likened to a tent at the end of camping season, once you've collapsed the pole; the canvas is left to drape loosely over whatever remains.

Early in my career, I treated one such individual. Anna P. first came to see me to discuss ways in which her sagging facial skin (the result of a 100-pound weight loss) could be tightened. Although, as I suspected, it was the same 100 pounds she had gained and lost countless times before, she assured me that this time the loss was permanent. Besides having maintained her current weight for close to four years, she said she now held an executive position with the weight-loss organization that had inspired her success and was under constant pressure there to stay thin. She felt the current state of her skin made her look a good twenty years older than she really was, and I agreed.

Several weeks following that first visit, Anna underwent a face lift. She was so pleased with the results of the cosmetic surgery that she went on to have a tummy tuck as well as liposuction in those few areas that exercise just wouldn't budge.

Today Anna looks like the daughter of the woman who originally came to see me. And although her life is now rich and rewarding in every way, she deeply regrets having spent the time and trouble she could have saved had she not subjected her body to such early abuse.

Heredity

It's been said that you can choose your friends but not your relatives. And since genetic composition is the single most determining factor when it comes to assessing the rate at which your skin will age, one look at your family can either make your hopes for maintaining a youthful complexion soar or send them plummeting into the depths of despair.

If your senior-citizen parents are constantly being mistaken for your second-grader's mom and dad, rejoice! You've probably inherited a wonderful set of genes. If, on the other hand, your folks looked like senior citizens even when *you* were in the second grade, don't fret, for all is not lost. You see, your "aging destiny" is, by no means, cast in iron. Rather, it happens to be quite flexible and capable of change.

By carefully nurturing and protecting the support structure of your body's largest organ, you will be able to hold back the signs of time in your skin for years to come and, in so doing, will change the course of (your family's aging) history!

CHANGES TO EXPECT AFTER THIRTY DAYS

Dry skin will begin to feel much more moist and less taut.

Surface facial wrinkles (such as those that commonly appear on the forehead, at the corners of the eyes, and between the nostrils and the sides of the mouth) will soften.

Feelings of lethargy will subside, replaced by a resurgence of energy.

Symptoms of insomnia will start to disappear; a general sense of well-being will be experienced.

The Second Thirty Days: Treating Special Problems

CHAPTER 10

ACNE

The person who started the rumor than acne was reserved for oily complexions obviously had a skintype other than dry. As anyone who has experienced it well knows, dry skin and acne are a formidable duo, and must be dealt with in a gingerly fashion if the treatment is to be deemed effective.

Unable to withstand the ultradrying side effects of the majority of topically applied medications, dry-skin acne is most effectively attacked from an internal standpoint, with mild external preparations employed for support.

My "strategic defense" plan begins with a little background material on your opponent, the world's most prevalent skin disease.

The "Family" of Acne Lesions

Definitely not the sort to which you'd willingly extend an invitation, the members of this clan are the kind that tend to show up uninvited. Before we proceed any further, I'd like to make you aware of the wide variety of forms this most unwelcome intruder can take.

How Acne Begins

The skin is made up of three layers: the subcutaneous layer (or fatty tissue); the dermis (which houses the blood vessels, nerves, sweat glands, and follicles); and the epidermis (which covers the dermis and serves as the skin's "overcoat"). Running through the dermis is the connective tissue that, as its name implies, is the supporting structure of the dermis.

While the sweat glands have a direct opening to the surface of the skin, the oil (or sebaceous) glands are not quite as fortunate. The oil (or sebum) produced in these glands must find its way to the skin's surface via a follicle or pore, some of which contain hair. This is where the trouble can get its start. If the cells that line these follicles stick together instead of sloughing off (as they do under normal conditions), acne begins, and all forms of acne initiate in the very same manner. Now for a closer look:

MICROCOMEDO. This earliest form of acne plug is not visible to the naked eye. Nonetheless, microcomedones are insidious and can (and often do) lead to more serious things.

CLOSED COMEDO. This more advanced stage of the microcomedo is also called a whitehead. Since there is almost no opening at the surface, the closed comedo must never be squeezed; in so doing, you would only force its contents deeper into the skin and run the risk of scarring.

OPEN COMEDO. Better known as the blackhead, the open comedo is an acne plug with an opening at the surface. Because of this fact, the contents of the blackhead can usually be emptied by exerting gentle pressure on both of its sides. (Be sure to first steam skin for 15 minutes.) Always use your index fingers, making sure they're wrapped with tissues before you start. (*NOTE*: Never use a "comedo extractor" to remove blackheads, as these instruments can do serious damage to the surrounding skin.) If the material does not come out easily, don't force it! Follow with a dab of 3% hydrogen peroxide on a cotton ball.

Blackheads are not caused by dirt. Their darkish color comes partially from the oxidation of the sebum and partially from the skin's own pigment or melanin. Therefore blackheads cannot simply be washed away.

PUSTULE. A small red bump that peaks with a yellowish cap of pus is known as a pustule. It is basically a comedo that has ruptured, and when this happens, your body's white blood cells rush in like the infantry to fight the "foreign invaders" which include bacteria, oil, and dead cells.

You may try to drain this type of acne lesion and, if properly done, this process will greatly accelerate the healing of the area. First, make sure your hands are scrupulously clean. Next, sterilize a needle by holding it in the flame of a match for a few seconds. After the needle has cooled, puncture the pustule in the exact center of the yellowish cap. With index fingers wrapped in tissue, gently squeeze the sides of the lesion. Stop when the pus no longer comes out easily. If you force it, you will drive the material deeper into the skin and greatly increase the likelihood of permanent scarring. Now place a warm compress (a clean washcloth soaked in warm water will do) over the area for a few minutes and finish by pressing with a cotton ball dipped in rubbing alcohol.

Warm-water soaks can and should be repeated several times daily until the lesion has healed. The warm water increases the flow of blood to the area and speeds up the healing process.

CYSTIC ACNE. If you have even one acne lesion that resembles a large boil or cyst, you should consider your condition severe and place yourself under the regular care of a qualified cosmetic dermatologist. If finances are worrying you, don't forget that most insurance companies cover acne treatments. Speak with your doctor.

My Step-by-step Method of Treatment

Mine is a multifactored approach to the treatment of acne. Although specific "routes" might vary slightly from patient to patient, in the end "all roads lead to Rome" (that is, clear skin).

STRESS. What better place to start than with a review of one of acne's primary aids and abetters—stress—and to reiterate the extremely detrimental effect it can have on skin. Have you ever experienced a breakout right before an unusually important event, perhaps your wedding or the start of a new job? It is the extra strain put on your emotions by these out-of-the-ordinary occasions that probably caused the blemishes to appear.

The chain of biological events that leads up to a breakout goes like this: Stress activates the hypothalamus gland, which in turn stimulates the pituitary gland. The pituitary sends a message to the adrenal gland indicating that a larger-than-normal number of male hormones (including androgen) should be released immediately. Androgen activates the oil glands to produce sebum, which can result in acne.

I've had cases in which excessive stress has caused patients to pick at blackheads so much that they've ended up creating serious cases of acne for themselves. And I've had one or two who didn't stop there, but went on to pick at the scab, causing permanent scarring.

Since a certain amount of stress is simply part of life, and is all right, the key to minimizing its adverse effects lies in the way we handle it. Learning to relax is the obvious solution, but very often this cannot be done by the individual acting alone. If, after thorough examination and testing, I feel that stress is at the root of the problem, I will suggest some form of psychological counseling to resolve the inner conflict.

EXERCISE. In more moderate cases of emotional stress (but ones that are clearly having an adverse effect on the skin), the addition of exercise to the daily routine may prove very beneficial. Not only does exercise stimulate the circulation and aid in the cleansing of the skin (by flushing out impurities through perspiration), it also reduces tension, thus improving one's mental outlook. And a positive outlook cannot be discounted when it comes to creating that "inner glow" so important to a beautiful complexion.

A few words of caution before you start, however. Since exercise does increase the activity of the sweat glands and a buildup of this perspiration can trap oils below the skin, you should always begin your regimen with a clean face and shower immediately after you're finished. Whenever possible, wear loose-fitting clothing while you work out, as chafing can aggravate acne on the back and chest. Finally, when selecting a form of exercise, it's wise to keep your choice in the "middle of the road" category— no marathons your first time out, please! Remember, too much of a good thing can sometimes be worse than nothing at all.

REST. Another important acne-combatant is adequate rest. Since the skin repairs and rejuvenates itself while we sleep, the importance of rest to a healthy complexion should be obvious. While needs tend to vary slightly from individual to individual, the standard eight hours per night should suffice for most. What's that you say? You can't possibly devote eight whole hours a day to *just sleeping*? Well, as the old saying goes, if it's really important, you'll find the time for it, and the proper amount of sleep is vital if you want to see an improvement in the condition of your skin.

DIET. "You are what you eat": In my opinion, these are some of the truest words ever spoken. Although the exact correlation between diet and acne remains something of a debate among doctors, I prefer to err on the side of caution. In compliance with this philosophy, I ask that you closely adhere to my basic nutritional program, as well as add the following acne aggravators to your "to be avoided" list:

> All dairy products
>
> Beef (because of the hormones given the animals to fatten them)
>
> Cabbage, shellfish, spinach, artichokes, iodized salt, and kelp (because of the high iodine content of these foods)

VITAMINS AGAINST ACNE. For maximum effectiveness, please incorporate these acne-fighting supplements into your daily vitamin-therapy regimen:

○ Vitamin A: 10,000 additional I.U.s (not to exceed 20,000 I.U.s without a doctor's supervision.)
○ Zinc: an extra 50 mg.
○ Lysine (an amino acid): 500 mg.

Finally, by increasing your daily intake of wheat germ by 2 tablespoons (from 1 to 3), you'll be providing your body with the additional vitamin F it needs to slow down your skin's production of oil.

Guidelines to Non-prescription and Prescription Drugs That Go to Work Immediately

Since acne starts when the cells that line the follicle stick together, instead of sloughing off as they normally do, one way to prevent the disease is to stop the cells from sticking together in the first place.

Fortunately, this can be accomplished. All you need is the proper drying-peeling agent for your skin type and a bit of knowledge regarding its correct usage. Drying-peeling agents work because they contain chemicals that get down *into* the follicle, unlike cleansers and astringents, to peel apart the dead cells that are trying to stick together. These products must be used with great regularity and must be rubbed into the skin.

In order for you to derive maximum benefits from your drying-peeling agent, it is essential that you choose one specifically formulated for your type of skin.

Because dry complexions can tolerate only the mildest of acne medications, choose from the three listed below to most effectively treat the disease in your skin:

Rezamid Acne Lotion

Fostex Medicated Cover-up

Clinique's Anti-Acne Formula (available in three shades)

Note: If even these preparations prove too harsh, while not drying-peeling agents, the following will dry and heal some blemishes.

Garlic (slice into thin wedges and squeeze the juice out with a garlic press directly onto blemish)

Lemon juice (freshly squeezed and dabbed directly onto the blemish using a cotton-tipped swab)

The juice of a raw Idaho potato (slice into thin wedges and squeeze the juice directly onto blemish)

Milk of magnesia (dabbed directly onto the blemish using a cotton-tipped swab)

THE PROCESS. Start by applying the drying-peeling agent to your face once a day, after washing. To avoid unnecessary irritation of the skin, make sure the area is completely dry before applying the medication (waiting 15 or 20 minutes). Cover areas that are currently broken out, as well as those that have a tendency to be. *But do not cover your entire face!* The T-zone (forehead, nose, and chin) is usually the prime spot for acne, but be sure to avoid placing the medication around the eyes and corners of the mouth, as these areas are much too sensitive for this type of treatment.

IS THE MEDICATION WORKING? You will know if you observe the surface peeling of your skin. Although your skin will appear slightly dry, this drying and peeling action will in no way harm your skin, nor will it cause wrinkles. The only thing you might find discouraging after you start your treatment is the possible appearance of new acne lesions. Believe me when I say that these would have shown up sooner or later. They stem from existing microcomedones, and the peeling action simply brought them to a head a little sooner than would have happened naturally. Remember, the important thing is to prevent new acne plugs from forming.

If your skin appears to be slightly reddened by the use of any acne medication, try applying one of the over-the-counter hydrocortisone cremes to the affected area: Cortaid or Lanacord, for example. This should be done after your drying-peeling agent has dried. The anti-inflammatory properties of these preparations should help to alleviate any minor irritation.

If your skin stops peeling or if your acne gets worse, you may have to alter your plan of action. Sometimes you need to strengthen your acne medication, which can be done in one of two ways: by increasing either the frequency of treatments or the strength of the drying-peeling agent. Never do both at the same time, thinking that if some is good, more is better. It isn't! You will know the change is working when peeling resumes. If the opposite is the case, that is, your medication seems to be too strong, take the reverse tack of decreasing either the frequency of treatments or the strength of the drying-peeling agent.

WINDING DOWN. After your acne has been under control for a period of four to eight weeks, you can begin a maintenance program. Once again, proceed with caution. Change one factor, proceeding one step at a time. Decrease the strength of the peeling agent or, if your acne was severe and you applied your medication twice a day, decrease it to just once. Remain at the lower level for at least two weeks before decreasing another step. Continue this downward progression until your face no longer peels. But

My Ninety-Day Plan for Dry Skin

if your acne flares up after you decrease your treatment, resume the level at which the condition was under control. Maintain that level until you once again feel confident enough to begin a "slow descent."

RETIN A(VITAMIN A ACID). One drying-peeling agent that requires a prescription is Retin A (tretinoin or retinoic acid, as it's sometimes known). Although the vast majority of acne sufferers will peel with an over-the-counter drying-peeling agent, there are some who will not. For these individuals, vitamin A acid can prove very effective in the clearing of the skin. But, as with any powerful drug, vitamin A acid is not without adverse side effects. Its usage may bring about intense surface peeling as well as extreme irritation in the skin of the patient who applies it too often or incorrectly. For this reason, I insist on close medical supervision of every individual engaged in this form of therapy.

Recently, Retin A has also proven an effective tool in the treatment of aging skin. While it is by no means a replacement for dermabrasion or the chemical peel, it will, through consistent usage, reverse some signs of photoaging (sun damage to the skin which causes premature aging) as well as minimize fine lines and wrinkles but must be used under medical supervision.

ACCUTANE. Another derivative of vitamin A used to treat very severe cases of cystic acne is the prescription drug accutane. Although touted by some as a wonder drug in treating difficult cases, my opinion is that dangers from the immediate (and unknown long-term) side effects brought on by the drug's usage, do outweigh its possible advantages. Of course, there is always the exception to the rule, but treatment with accutane is something I prescribe only as a last resort. Here are some of the reasons why: The most serious side effect produced by accutane is the documented fact that it can cause birth defects in unborn fetuses. Any woman of childbearing age who is contemplating using the drug should therefore submit to a pregnancy test and be carefully monitored by her doctor throughout the duration of treatment. In addition, accutane frequently causes excessively dry lips, nosebleeds, elevated lipid levels, pains and swelling in the joints and occasional personality changes. Still, as it is sometimes the only thing that will bring really stubborn cases of acne under control, the afflicted individual is often willing to take the risks. Accutane is taken by mouth and the blood must be frequently monitored.

ANTIBIOTICS. The most widely prescribed antibiotic in the treatment of acne is tetracycline, which works by effecting the creation of fatty acids within the follicle. The most common side effect of taking tetracycline is the yeast infection it seems to produce in certain women (a risk that can be minimized by adding two extra tablespoons of acidophilus to your daily "beauty cocktail"). Photosensitivity can also be a problem for some people, and tetracycline should be discontinued when going into the sun. If you are taking a multivitamin while on tetracycline, make sure it is a formula that does not contain iron, as that mineral blocks the body's absorption of the drug, and avoid milk products.

If tetracycline ceases to be effective in controlling a patient's acne, the doctor will often switch to erythromycin, an antibiotic that works in much the same way. Minocycline is a chemical derivative of tetracycline that has proven effective in some instances when plain tetracycline has failed. The side effects that accompany minocycline can be more severe than those experienced through the usage of tetracycline; one side effect is dizziness.

Sometimes such antibiotics as tetracycline, erythromycin, clindamycin, and lincomycin are used in topical applications with excellent results. The main advantage of a topical over a systemic medicine (one which enters the system) is in the reduced instances of side effects.

BIRTH CONTROL PILLS. When birth control pills were first introduced nearly thirty years ago, they contained very large doses of estrogen and almost always contributed to an improved complexion in acne sufferers. But since estrogens also generated many undesirable side effects, pharmaceutical manufacturers began introducing pills that were formulated with greatly reduced amounts of the hormone. Although these newer pills are easier for most women to take, they do not provide the same degree of relief from acne as did their predecessors. In fact, some formulations may even make the condition worse.

Birth control pills generally thought to help acne are Demulen, Enovid-E, Enovid-5, and Ovulen. Those that usually aggravate the disease include Norinyl, Norlestrin, Ortho-Novum, and Ovral. If you are currently taking one of the formulas believed to worsen acne, speak with your doctor about a possible change in your prescription. (Don't forget to take B-complex vitamins when taking birth control pills.)

INTRALESIONAL STEROID SHOTS. The times during when I've felt a kinship to my fellow physicians the obstetricians are the times when I've had a model, actress, or other highly visible individual rushed into my office so that I might administer the "magical injection" that would deliver her to an impending photo shoot or TV commercial, blemish-free. (Fortunately, I've never been called out in the middle of the night for this!) These shots contain a dosage of corticosteroids that is injected directly into the acne lesion. Because the anti-inflammatory properties of cortisone rapidly shrink the blemish, it is usually gone within a couple of days. Occasional dimpling or depression in the skin can occur secondary to these intralesional steroid injections, but fortunately this dimpling is usually reversible and transitory.

Acne Scars Don't Have to Be Forever

I would be greatly remiss to conclude this section without mentioning the wide variety of cosmetic surgery procedures now available to aid in the correction of acne scars. Although I will explain each in the section devoted to cosmetic surgery, I can assure you that there is no need to wear the scars obtained in the heat of your battle with acne. Thanks to the many advances of modern technology, there are several very viable means for virtually eliminating them so that, in the end, "all that's left is the memory." Fortunately for acne sufferers, memories (unlike scars) do tend to fade completely with time!

DRY SENSITIVE SKIN

If calming your sensitive skin reads like a scene from *The Taming of the Shrew*, I'd like to offer the following very comforting solutions:

> Before using any new product on your skin (cleanser, moisturizer, or makeup), always patch-test it first by applying a small amount to your forearm. Allow it to

remain undisturbed for a period of 24 hours. If no irritation develops, you can consider the product safe and proceed with its usage. If, however, any redness or swelling appears in the area, discard the remainder of product and write its purchase price off to experience. (You might be financially wiser to always rely on in-store testers for this purpose.)

Be sure to wash bed linens, face cloths, towels, and any items of personal clothing in a mild, low-sudsing soap such as Ivory. Avoid at all costs regular detergents (which tend to leave a residue) as well as any other harsh products that may come in contact with your skin. If *total* avoidance is simply not possible (when cleaning, for example), protect yourself by wearing rubber gloves.

Never use tissues (such as Kleenex) to remove makeup (or for any other purpose) on your face. They contain fine wood shavings that can easily scratch and irritate delicate skin. Pads of cotton are a much safer alternative.

For facial cleansing, always be sure to use cloths made of 100 percent cotton. You can easily make these yourself by purchasing a package of cloth diapers and cutting them into squares of four. These cloths double as very convenient and soothing masks, if two pieces are alternately dipped in a basin of ice water to which a couple of drops of vinegar have been added. Allow one to rest on your face until the chill has worn off, and then switch to the other piece. Keep doing this for 15 to 20 minutes to calm redness or irritation.

Use extra caution when bleaching or waxing facial hair, as this delicate area is very suseptible to problems. To be on the safe side, have it done professionally.

Last but not least, remember to handle your skin as little as possible. Don't rub your face vigorously, and above all, don't scratch it! If itching occurs, place an ice cube in a handkerchief and apply to the area of itching for five or six seconds. The itching will stop!

My Ninety-Day Plan for Dry Skin

SKIN DURING PREGNANCY AND MENOPAUSE

Pregnancy and the Dry Skin

Although, because of an increased production of oil, dry skin generally flourishes during the early months of pregnancy (a small compensation for morning sickness), the latter half finds it once again its old taut self. The negative effects of hormonally induced dryness can, however, be kept to a minimum, simply through increased awareness.

Once you're prepared for what's in store and are ready to treat your skin accordingly, by adding moisture whenever and wherever it's needed, you can maintain a complexion that's glowing for the full nine months!

Menopause

Unless estrogen therapy is employed, dry skin is known to mature rather badly. However, this is a totally preventable phenomenon if the guidelines of my anti-aging plan are closely adhered to. If you stick by it, it will do the same for you. It's also not a bad idea to increase your moisturizing wherever necessary.

Because the symptoms of menopause can range from slightly uncomfortable to downright hair-raising, some doctors have a tendency to overprescribe (i.e. tranquilizers, sleeping pills, anti-anxiety, anti depressant drugs—all potentially habit forming) in an effort to help their patients cope. Bear in mind that *any* medication can have an adverse effect on skin. Before taking it, always weigh the odds. A brisk 30-minute walk each day can do wonders for your state of mind (not to mention your body), so before submitting to chemical mood alteration (i.e. drugs), why not give the physical approach a try by making regular aerobic exercise (jogging, swimming, biking or walking) an integral part of your life.

CHANGES TO EXPECT AFTER SIXTY DAYS

Dry skin should be much less so now with scaly patches virtually non-existent.

Your eyes should be sparkling at this point with the whites appearing much clearer.

Any sign of insomnia will have vanished by now, enabling you to have a good night's rest every night!

CHAPTER 11

The Third Thirty Days: Completing the Plan

BODY CARE

You'll find that the skin on your body derives the same positive effects from my anti-aging plan as the skin on your face.

Hands and Feet

Two areas are always a source of concern, regardless of one's skintype: the hands and the feet. For this reason, I'd like to provide you with an overview of preventative care for each.

Over the years, I've seen hundreds of women spend thousands of dollars in an effort to preserve the fresh-faced look of a girl of 25. But a problem occurs when the hands dangling out of their sleeves are decidedly those of a 50-year-old matron. For this reason, if a patient is undergoing a facial cosmetic surgery procedure, I will frequently suggest a hand procedure as well.

Unless you are prepared to wear gloves every day for the rest of your life, don't let your hands "give you away." If you follow these simple suggestions, that will never happen:

Keep a bottle of moisturizer next to each sink in your home, and apply it to your hands after every washing.

Wear cotton-lined rubber gloves when submerging your hands in water. A pair of plain white (dyes are potential irritants to the skin) cotton gloves may be worn under regular rubber gloves.

To prevent ugly brown spots from appearing, be sure to include your hands when applying daily sunscreen one half hour before going in the sun. And when temperatures dictate the need for a coat, wear gloves as well.

Hands can also benefit from the masks you use on your face.

Keep your nails neatly manicured; they can be a distinct beauty asset, or a liability if neglected.

Try massaging an antiperspirant into sweaty palms. This should help to alleviate any potential embarrassment. If you find it irritating, consult your doctor, as there is a new process called ionophoresis that is effective.

Apply moisturizer to hands before going to bed, and, if they're feeling particularly rough and chapped, "lock it in" by wrapping them in a layer of Saran Wrap covered by a pair of white cotton gloves. The slight discomfort involved in this procedure is well worth the results it produces.

Our feet really take a beating each day, which is why nature provided us with an extra thick protective sole. However, if left unattended, the skin in this area becomes extremely thick, tough, and generally unattractive. Regularity of care is the key to prevent this from happening. If you follow these simple guidelines every day, your feet will keep you "walking on air" for the rest of your life:

At the end of the day, fill a small plastic basin with warm soapy water (you may prefer to use bath oil) and give your feet a good soak for at least 15 minutes (longer, if time permits).

Pat dry and go over any rough, calloused areas (such as heels) with a pumice stone. For stubborn callouses, try standing in an inch or two of bleach, which will have a softening effect. Pat dry after one minute and apply a good moisturizer.

Lavish with moisturizer and, one night a week (more if you wish), wrap your feet in Saran Wrap, as suggested for the hands, substituting white cotton socks for gloves.

It's also an excellent idea to prop your legs up with a couple of pillows and relax for 20 minutes each day. This reverses the pull of gravity your feet and legs are constantly exposed to and gives them a much-needed "breather."

Finally, be sure to change shoes, from high heels to low, very often. This relieves the calf muscles and keeps the Achilles tendon from becoming shortened.

Acne on the Back

Acne on the back is a frequent complaint. It seems to affect a wide cross-section of individuals of all skintypes. Here's the best way for everyone to bring it under control:

Always use a back brush and mild soap to properly cleanse the area during your daily shower or bath.

After the area is thoroughly dry, apply a slightly stronger drying-peeling agent (say 10 percent benzoyl peroxide) than you'd use on your face. This suggestion is made because of the difficulty involved in reapplication of the product. (Thorough coverage of the area requires the aid of another person. If you live alone, just do the best that you can.)

Since it is not necessary to wash the area before the drying-peeling agent is applied, apply it once in the morning and once before retiring.

If the acne on your back is very severe, it may be necessary for you to add another bath or shower to your daily routine, at least until the condition has been brought under control. (Don't forget to remoisturize dry areas of the body immediately afterwards.)

Finally, if all of your attempts to bring the condition under control fail, consult a dermatologist before scarring occurs. Some problems of this nature are very stubborn and will respond only to prescription-strength medication.

Warning: These Ingredients May Be Hazardous to the Health of Your Skin

The following is a list of potential irritants to dry skin found in treatment products, moisturizers and foundations. Although they may not bother you now, skins do change. For this reason, always check the label of every new product before you buy it, particularly if your skin is feeling especially sensitive.

○ Camphor
○ Menthol
○ Talc
○ Alcohol
○ Magnesium aluminum silicate
○ Detergent-based cleansers
○ Fragrance

SUN SPECIFICS

Aging's first lieutenant in the field, the sun is beauty's greatest natural enemy. Although total avoidance is your only secure defense, it would be difficult to imagine a life lived entirely on the "inside." In lieu of that approach, here are some of the most effective ways I've found to minimize the effects of the sun:

Get into the sunscreen habit. Apply one with an SPF of at least 15 every morning, alone or under makeup one half hour before exposure to the sun. (With SPF 15 protection, the skin can tolerate the sun 15 times longer than without a protective product. With SPF 4, 4 times longer, etc.) I believe sunscreen of SPF 15 or 20 is about the most effective you can get today. More than that is just wishful thinking.

To protect the areas that are among the first to show signs of aging, always include hands and neck in your sunscreen coverage.

Because the skin on your lips contains very little melanin, this area requires SPF protection of its own. Make sure it gets it by regularly using one of the "lip blocks" on the market, either alone or under your lipstick. (The brighter the shade, the better the protection.) Remember to reapply frequently whenever you're out in the sun, and always after eating or drinking.

Don't forget your sunglasses. Wear them twelve months of the year! Best are the wraparound kind and ones that indicate their UV (Ultra Violet) protection. To further shield this delicate area, use one of the sunblocks created specifically for use around eyes.

Hats (especially the wide-brimmed variety) are always in style when it comes to spending a day in the sun.

Avoid taking PABA by mouth. Taken orally, it frequently incites a negative reaction in the skin.

Don't believe the ads: Sun beds and tanning booths are every bit as detrimental to skin as the real thing.

All of the following can make you extrasensitive to sun. If you must be in it, avoid them:

Many medications, including antibiotics, birth control pills, diuretics, and tranquilizers. Check with your doctor to see if anything else you might be taking applies.

Germicidal soaps and antiseptics that contain hexachlorophene and bithionol.

Any product that's alcohol based, such as astringent, perfume, after-shave, and cologne.

Excessive amounts of vitamins A and C.

Remember: *Be afraid of your own shadow*! It's there to remind you that the sun's damaging rays are lurking close by.

CHANGES TO EXPECT AFTER NINETY DAYS

You should feel as though you're wearing someone else's skin, and the trade was definitely made in *your* favor!

Your surface facial wrinkles should have all but disappeared, making you look substantially younger than you did a short three months ago.

Your energy level will be at an all-time high. You'll feel totally alert and on top of the world!

147

Saving Face (and More) Via Cosmetic Surgery and Dermatology

PART IV

Japanese culture dictates that to "lose face" (that is, to surrender one's dignity in disgrace) is to suffer the ultimate loss. Within that society, the preservation of personal honor is of paramount importance. Are our values and priorities so different? What do any of us really strive for, if not to maintain our individual senses of integrity and self-esteem?

A significant contributing factor to a woman's perception of her self-worth is her appearance: not only the way in which she is viewed by others but, more importantly, the way in which she appears to herself. If, for example, she is dismayed by something she sees (or doesn't see) in the mirror each morning, her ability to perform at optimum level throughout the day cannot help but be undermined.

Suppose we could change the things we find bothersome about our appearance and, hence, enhance the way we look. Would this not serve to enhance the way we feel about ourselves and others, too? Thanks to the many advances and discoveries made in recent years in the field of cosmetic surgery, that possibility can, to a great extent, become reality. Perhaps the most exciting discovery of all, however, will come with the realization that the "you" in your mind's eye can become the "you" that the rest of the world sees.

If living well is the best revenge, cosmetic surgery and dermatology can only serve to make it better, along with offering a renewed sense of hope to those who've "fallen down" along the way. Choose a doctor who will have both medical and surgical modalities to treat you. Remember, there are many conditions that can be treated cosmetically without surgery. And above all, feel comfortable with your doctor.

Here, then, are the categories of problems I most frequently face, along with the options available for solving each.

Procedures that Renew the Skin

CHAPTER 12

FOR THE RESURFACING OF SKIN

Chemical Peel

Legend has it that the first facial peels were self-induced by courtesans who, driven by the desire to stay young, would graze their faces over an open flame, thus burning the top layers of skin. Fortunately, medical science has come a long way since the days when this primitive forerunner of the chemical peel was performed! In fact, recent studies have shown that today's chemical peel, if correctly administered, can have effects beyond such relatively immediate ones as the smoothing of fine wrinkles, lines, superficial acne scars, and age spots. It's been demonstrated that even up to twenty years after the peel was performed, the skin that received the treatment is healthier, in structure and appearance, than the same individual's skin that was not peeled.

Here's how it's done: A solution of caustic chemicals (usually phenol or trichloracetic acid) is carefully painted onto the skin—either over the entire face or just on select spots—causing a chemical burn to the treated area. Immediately thereafter, the raw and oozing skin is sometimes covered with a waterproof tape that enhances the peel depending on the doctor's preference. After a couple of days, the tape is removed, and the doctor applies a medicated drying agent that rapidly induces the formation of a scab. When the scab falls off, in another week or so, the skin is very pink and extremely sensitive to sun. For this reason, I advise my patients to totally avoid exposure to the sun for at least a month and to wear a sunblock with an SPF of 15 for an additional six to eight months following the procedure.

Milder versions of the chemical peel can also be performed by mixing a lower concentration of the caustic chemical in the solution that is painted on. These beneficial "booster" or touch up peels are a regular part of my ongoing rejuvenation program. Sometimes these latter type of peels plus my home regimen will suffice.

Dermabrasion

A standard procedure in the treatment of acne scars, dermabrasion is often preferred by doctors over the chemical peel because of the extreme accuracy it affords them in abrading the skin. It is accomplished as follows: First, the patient is given a relaxant IV (one containing a sedative such as Valium to relax the patient), and then, to further minimize discomfort, six sites on the face are injected with an anesthetic. Next, the area to be dermabraded* (the whole face or just specific spots) is frozen with a refrigerant spray and mechanically resurfaced via the use of a high-speed wire or diamond-edged brush. Once again, the treated skin is raw and oozing immediately after the procedure and will form a scab. The healing time is similar to that following the chemical peel, but a few precautions regarding dermabrasion should be cited.

One of the major drawbacks of the procedure is that it can result in hyper- or hypopigmentation (an increase or decrease in the amount of color in the skin), primarily the latter. This problem should be of special concern to women with dark or olive complexions, as it is in individuals with this skintone that the problem usually arises. Because this condition can also be induced by some types of oral contraceptives, birth control pills may have to be discontinued for several weeks before and after surgery. Again, the skin will remain pink and very vulnerable to sunburn for several months following the dermabrasion and must be protected.

---

*Like the chemical peel, this can entail the whole face or just specific spots. This spot method can be "tricky," however.

Chemodermabrasion

I am one of the pioneers in the development of this progressive procedure, and I have given lectures world-wide about my findings, most recently at the International Society of Aesthetic Surgery in Tokyo and at the Italian Society of Aesthetic Surgery in Rome. Chemodermabrasion can, in many cases, prove to be the best of both worlds. Marrying the two traditional skin-resurfacing techniques (the dermabrasion is performed first, followed by the chemical peel, used in varying concentrations, depending on the skin type) provides for their mutual enhancement and, in many patients, can produce optimum results. Healing time and follow-up are about the same as for the other two procedures. I have found the results to be so superior that I almost always combine chemical peeling with dermabrading.

If scarring or "ice-pick" scars are present, usually "punch grafts" or punch elevation is performed before the chemodermabrasion. The chemodermabrasion is then performed 4–6 weeks later. In rare instances, a second chemodermabrasion may be necessary after sufficient time has been allowed for the skin to heal completely.

BEFORE

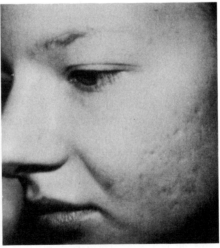

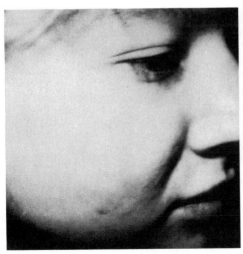

AFTER

FOR ''FILLING IN'' ACNE SCARS AND WRINKLES

Zyderm Collagen Injections

As the first physician on the East Coast to employ the use of injectable collagen* in the treatment and correction of such facial skin depressions as fine lines and superficial acne scars, I remain today (after successfully utilizing the material in well over 2,000 patients), a leading proponent of the substance's ability to best accomplish this task. Unlike synthetic silicone** (used by some doctors for a similar purpose), collagen is derived from a natural protein that, after implantation directly into the skin's concavity, provides a framework to which the body's newly produced cells and blood vessels can adhere. In addition, the latest collagen derivative, Zyplast, has proven very effective in the ''erasing'' of heavier facial lines and creases as well as in certain reconstructive procedures involving the cheeks and chin. It does not tend to be absorbed into the patient's system as rapidly as Zyderm, making the use of this third-generation*** collagen often preferable.

Because once injected the substance becomes part of the body's ever-changing system, collagen must be periodically† readministered if its results are to last. Another caution regarding collagen injections is the precision with which they must be placed in the skin's layers. The physician's innate skill and degree of advanced training in the area are therefore crucial in the successful administration of this very tricky technique.

Since approximately 1 percent‡ of those seeking collagen therapy have shown some evidence of an allergic reaction to the substance, all those wishing to undergo its treatments must first have a small amount of the material injected into the inner portion

---

*This term in no way refers to the collagen that is topically applied, as the substance in this form makes absolutely no change in the skin's structure.

**Liquid silicone has never been medically approved for the purpose of filling in skin imperfections. Additionally, the substance has been known to shift positions within the layers of skin into which it was injected.

***Zyplast Collagen was preceded by Zyderm Collagen I and II.

†The absorption rate of collagen depends to a great extent on the individual system of the patient undergoing its therapy and the area into which it is injected. But generally speaking, it must be ''touched up'' every six months to two years.

‡Especially susceptible are individuals with a family history of an autoimmune disease such as lupus or rheumatoid arthritis.

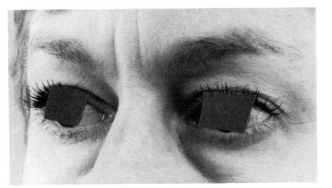

*Saving Face
(and More)
via Cosmetic
Surgery and
Dermatology*

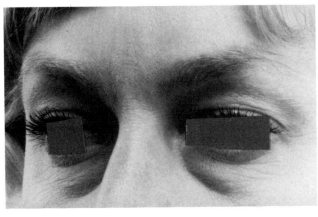

AFTER

BEFORE AFTER

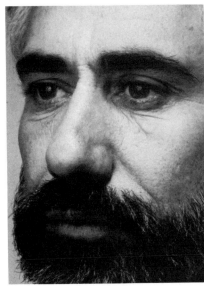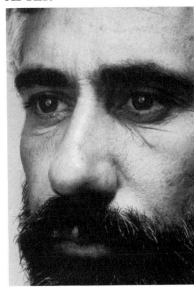

of their forearm. If after thirty days no undue irritation develops, the patient can proceed as planned. However, even an adverse reaction does not mean that all hope is lost, for doctors have recently developed a viable alternative to collagen injections: fat cell transplantation surgery, or microlipotransfer.

Microlipotransfer

The latest procedural breakthrough for the filling in of facial skin depressions, microlipotransfer (or fat-cell transplantation surgery) was first performed in Europe. This technique utilizes tiny transplants of fat cells harvested from the patient's abdomen or hips, combined with distilled water to create collagen, for injection into deep-seated facial furrows and contour deformities. It has proven most effective. An anesthetic is required, and this technique is best suited for large defects or atrophy in the face and body. *So far* no complications have been reported. Because of the newness of the procedure, however, it has yet to be determined exactly how long its results will last, but it is a graft and no other allergic reaction is possible since it is the patient's own tissue.

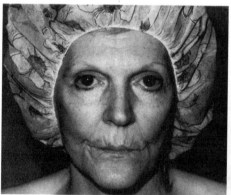

BEFORE

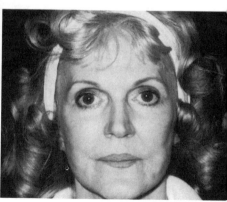

AFTER

Autologous Regeneration Therapy

As I've mentioned, it's my opinion that face lifts are performed more frequently than necessary. When a balloon starts to lose air, would you stretch the balloon's skin even tighter to fix it, or would you put more air into the balloon? Surgery should be performed on the content, not the container! As people age, they lose fat under the skin; there is of course some laxity of the skin also. My concept of Autologous Regeneration Therapy (A.R.T.), is simple, straightforward, and not as costly as a face lift. I simply take the patient's own fat through the process of microlipotransfer and redistribute it to the "three pillars of the face," the two cheekbones and the area around the mouth, with simple injections, in the same manner as collagen injections are used to alleviate wrinkles. You can prove to yourself how effective this can be with this simple test: Smile in front of a mirror, a big grin. Look how healthy and youthful your face becomes! You have just simply pushed fat up into the cheekbone area. It is this that makes one look younger, not tightening the skin!

Surgical Excision of Scars

As previously mentioned, due to the irregular shape or depth of certain scars (acne or otherwise), their correction is often best achieved by means of either incising the area with a scalpel or by "punching it out" with a small cylindrical knife. Known as a biopsy punch, that performs much like a cookie cutter, and then stitching the surrounding skin thereby is grafted back together. This type of procedure is especially effective on "ice pick" acne scars.

Cosmetic Concealment

For nonsurgical help in camouflaging acne's ravages or wrinkling of the skin prior to or when not opting for cosmetic surgery, here's a rundown of what's available in the way of concealment via cosmetics. It should be noted that the effects obtainable through the usage of these products are temporary, at best.

GREEN-TONED PRIMERS. When worn under foundation, these formulas are able, to a certain degree, to neutralize the redness of the skin that acne scars can cause. Use them only where necessary and, if acne is still active or your skin is very oily, avoid formulas with a moisturing base. Two examples are Stendhal's Soin Bio-rosis (for dry or sensitive skin), and Madeline Mono's water-based foundation in Aqua (for oily or combination skins).

SKIN REFINERS. Based on the premise that light reflects, this fairly innovative category of products, when applied sparingly to skin depressions (scars or wrinkles), acts to draw light to the area, thus creating the illusion of a smoother, more even surface. Two examples are Estée Lauder's Lightworks Color Balancer and Clinique's Zero Base, both of which can be worn on bare skin or under or over makeup.

PORE MINIMIZERS. Usually a type of oil-free foundation, pore minimizers do tend to provide for a diminished look in the size of the pores. Since they often contain a form of powder, they must be shaken very well prior to application. Generally most effective on oily skins, examples are Elizabeth Arden's Extra Help Oil-Free Make-up and Janet Sartin's Astringent (tinted).

HEAVY CONCEALERS. Originally developed to conceal such noticeable problems as birthmarks and severe scarring from burns, these products (such as Lydia O'Leary's Covermark and Dermablend) may also help to conceal lesser insults to the skin. Lightly pat (*never* rub) concealer over the area in need of correction, after foundation, but before powder, has been applied.

CREASE FILLERS. Touted as spackle for the skin, these products (Line Filler by Adrien Arpel and Erase by Max Factor) are used prior to foundation, theoretically to even out the "cracks" (wrinkles, lines, and depressions) in one's complexion. Because of their heavy texture, however, they must be applied with a very light hand and allowed to dry for at least two or three minutes to avoid the "Cats" look—pseudo-whiskers that are the result of improper blending or too heavy application of corrective product.

Procedures that Reshape the Face and Body

CHAPTER 13

FOR THE "TAILORING" OF SAGGING SKIN

The Face Lift (Rhytidectomy)

Just as a seamstress or tailor can reshape a garment by taking necessary "nips and tucks," so the cosmetic surgeon can alter the contours of the facial skin, restoring it to the snug fit it had in its prime.* This tailoring is accomplished by means of the face lift, the procedure that has become the cornerstone of cosmetic surgery. While I do feel this operation is performed more frequently than necessary (especially on younger patients) the fact remains that for truly sagging skin, this is the only process that will be effective.

Although techniques vary to a certain degree among doctors, the most common (and safest) way to perform the face lift is by beginning an incision on the patient's scalp (well within the hairline), continuing down and under the earlobe, and ending behind the back of the ear. The skin is then lifted away from the underlying fat and pulled upward and backward, with any excess trimmed away at the line of incision. The remaining skin is carefully anchored down, and the opening is closed by means of fine sutures.

---

*The degree of success achieved through the face lift depends on a variety of patient factors (including heredity, degree of sun damage, and general condition of the skin), as well as the physician's skill.

The patient's head is wrapped in bandages that are removed within twenty-four hours.

Some swelling and discoloration of the skin will follow, but to what degree depends in large measure on each individual's reaction to the operation. Generally speaking, the patient can appear in public approximately three weeks following the face lift and should look better than ever three weeks after that. Some-

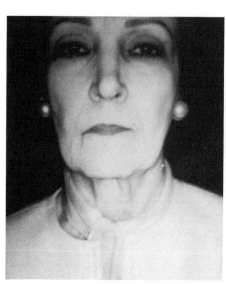

BEFORE

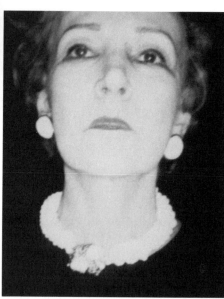

AFTER

times there is a peel or chemodermabrasion done around the lips at the time of the face lift. Many doctors perform liposuction surgery of the neck and a neck-lift at the time of the facelift.

The Eye Lift (Blepharoplasty)

An eye lift is accomplished by making a small incision in the upper eyelid. Through the incision, which is completely contained within the eyelid's crease, the surgeon removes all of the excess and overhanging skin that has been plaguing the area and possibly obscuring the vision. At this time, some skin, muscle, and fat are removed. The opening is then closed by means of extra fine sutures.

The scar that results is generally imperceptible, because of its location in the fold of the eyelid.

A correction in the lower lid is accomplished by making an incision just below the eyelash line and lifting the skin up from the underlying tissue. Part of the cushioning fat pads are removed from their compartments below the eye as well as some skin, muscle and fat. The freed skin is then drawn upward, and the

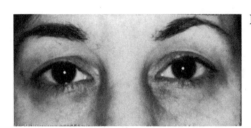

BEFORE

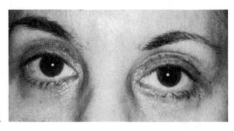

AFTER

resulting excess is removed very carefully. As with the upper lid, the incision is closed with very fine sutures and, once again, the ensuing scar will be practically invisible. Because of the structure of the lower lid, it may not be possible to eliminate all wrinkles by means of this procedure. Further enhancement of the area may be achieved by a form of the chemical peel.

If fat is a problem (typically with younger patients), a visible scar can be completely avoided by doing a transconjunctival approach. This involves making an incision in the sac between the eyeball and the inner skin of the lid called conjunctia. Fat is removed in this manner with minimal trauma and is an excellent modality when indicated.

Lip Augmentation

A frequent request from patients with thin lips is a fuller, more sensual look. This can be accomplished by injecting medically pure silicone, collagen, or the patient's own fat. The procedure is almost painless, and is usually found quite appealing.

FOR RECONTOURING THE FACE

Cheek Implant (Malar Implant)

For those with long and narrow faces, cheek implants can provide the much-desired "high-fashion" look. A relatively simple office procedure usually performed under local anesthesia (usually with preoperative sedation), solid plastic implants are inserted through the mouth to add prominence and projection to the patient's own cheekbones. The results are often very dramatic, once the initial swelling subsides (in three to five days). Bruising is minimal, and the patient can return to work in eight to ten days.

For those patients who don't want actual implants, it is possible

BEFORE

AFTER

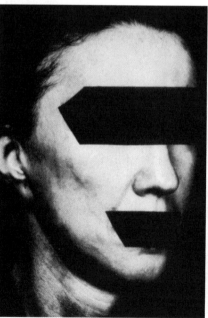
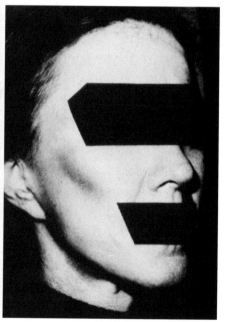

to inject the patient's own fat, or occasionally collagen, directly into the cheek area.

Chin Implant (Augmentation Mentoplasty)

To correct a receded or "weak" chin, I perform what is known as an augmentation mentoplasty, or chin implant. Done in the office or in the operating room and with general or local anes-

BEFORE

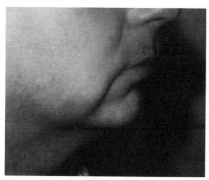

AFTER

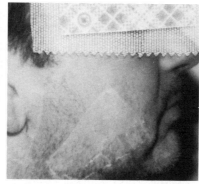

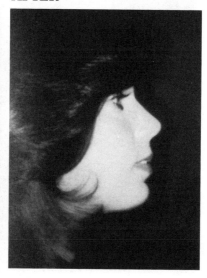

BEFORE

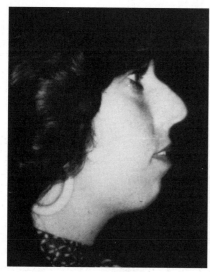

AFTER

thesia (usually with preoperative sedation), a solid plastic implant is inserted through an incision under the chin. Sometimes the implant is inserted through the mouth, thus requiring no outside incision. Tape placed over the chin to anchor the new implant should be left in place for five to seven days. Internal sutures dissolve and need not be removed. And external "skin" sutures are removed within five to seven days.

Swelling usually subsides within ten days and, if any bruising does occur, it's usually under the chin. The patient can easily return to work in eight to ten days.

Liposuction surgery of the chin and jawbone area is also frequently performed from the same incision. Occasionally, fat injections can be performed in the chin area as well.

FOR BODY REALIGNMENT

Liposuction (Suction Lipectomy)

To permanently remove stubborn deposits of fat that have refused to budge through dieting and exercise, liposuction can prove a very beneficial procedure. Performed in the office or hospital un-

BEFORE

AFTER

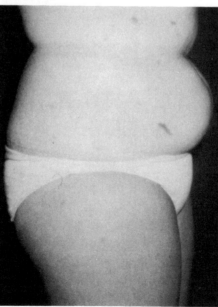
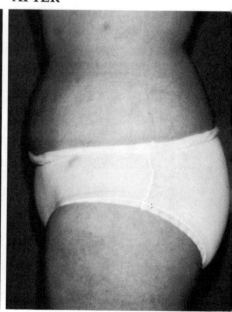

der either a local or general anesthesia (depending on the size of the area involved), the fat is literally vacuumed out of the body by means of a suction tube inserted through a tiny incision that is subsequently stitched closed.

Support bandages and a girdle are worn for five to ten days, and stitches are removed in approximately a week. Initial discomfort rapidly subsides (usually within two days), and most patients are very pleased with the results.

If any of our readers would like more information about Dr. Feder—his treatments, his services or the more than ninety products that he manufactures and dispenses for his patients, please feel free to write to Dr. Feder for a free brochure at:

Lewis M. Feder, M.D.
965 Fifth Avenue
New York, NY 10021
212-535-8700

Please enclose a self-addressed, stamped envelope.

In addition, Dr. Feder has produced the first cosmetic videotape (VHS), which is a one hour long informative film on different procedures, costs, and pros and cons. This tape is $29.95, plus $3.00 postage and handling.

Dr. Feder is also pleased to announce the formation of "Dr. Feder's Beauty and Skin Club." If you would like to be kept on our mailing list, please write to us.